Understanding the Nursing Process

Understanding the Nursing Process

SECOND EDITION

Leslie D. Atkinson, R.N., M.S.
Instructor, Nursing Program
Normandale Community College
Bloomington, Minnesota

Mary Ellen Murray, R.N., M.S.
Formerly Director, Nursing Program
Normandale Community College
Bloomington, Minnesota

Illustrated by Mark Atkinson

Macmillan Publishing Co., Inc.
NEW YORK

Collier Macmillan Canada, Inc.
TORONTO

Collier Macmillan Publishers
LONDON

Earlier edition entitled *Understanding the Nursing Process*
by Leslie D. Atkinson and Mary Ellen Murray

copyright © 1980 by Macmillan Publishing Co., Inc.

Macmillan Publishing Co., Inc.
866 Third Avenue, New York, New York 10022

Collier Macmillan Canada, Inc.
Collier Macmillan Publishers • London

Printing: 3 4 5 6 7 8 9   Year: 3 4 5 6 7 8 9 0 1

Library of Congress Cataloging in Publication Data

Atkinson, Leslie D.
  Understanding the nursing process.

  Bibliography: p.
  Includes index.
  1. Nursing.   I. Murray, Mary Ellen.   II. Title.
[DNLM: 1. Nursing process—Outlines. WY 18 A876u]
RT41.A82   1983   610.73   82-17255
ISBN 0-02-304580-9

Dedication
To Gary
To Peter

Preface to the Second Edition

In the years that followed the publication of the first edition of *Understanding the Nursing Process*, we have become increasingly aware of the necessity and professional responsibility for writing clear and complete nursing care plans. Several trends within health care provision which contributed to this awareness are:

1. Entry into independent practice of professional nurses
2. Increasing scope of independent nursing actions
3. Increasing acuity levels of hospitalized patients
4. Increasing legal accountability of nurses for nursing practice
5. Institutional quality of care standards which require that each patient has a documented care plan within 24 hours of admission
6. Institutional policies which require nursing care plans be retained as part of patient's permanent records
7. Development of the registered nurse licensing examination based on the nursing process steps of: assessing, analyzing, planning, implementing, and evaluating

While we recognize the five steps of the nursing process used in the revised licensing examination for registered nurses, this text retains the four-step nursing process format: assessing, planning, implementing, and evaluating. The activities identified within the analysis step as described by the National Council of State Boards of Nursing are clearly described within the assessment and planning chapters of this book.

The fifth step of analysis was added to reduce the amount of overlap within testing categories and to further separate nursing behaviors for the licensing examination. We believe that for instructional clarity and simplicity, the determination of both short- and long-term goals is more an act of synthesis than analysis and choose to retain this activity and related content within the planning step of the nursing process.

This edition will again emphasize a pragmatic approach to writing nursing care plans. The application of the nursing process is viewed as a nursing skill requiring practice and development. Other features of this text include:

1. An introduction designed to help the student understand the process and value its use
2. Four chapters corresponding to the four steps of the nursing process: assessment, planning, implementation, evaluation
3. Definitions, illustrations, and practice exercises related to the four steps of the nursing process
4. Definitions enclosed in boxes that stand out from the body of the text
5. Application of teaching–learning principles within the care-planning process
6. An appendix which consists of 11 care plans spanning growth and development levels from infancy to old age
7. A writing style with illustrations which is designed to make the book more enjoyable

Finally, we wish to acknowledge the sample nursing care plans contributed by Tom Olson and Rebecca Dunning, Normandale nursing faculty members whose expertise enhanced this aspect of the text, and to Ann Becker of the National Group for Classification of Nursing Diagnoses who granted permission to reproduce the classification of nursing diagnoses included in the text. Thank you also to other faculty members, to our students, and to the nursing staff of Bethesda North Hospital of Cincinnati, Ohio, all of whom helped to challenge our thinking and to continue the development of the nursing process.

L. D. A.

M. E. M.

Contents

Appendix: Sample Nursing Care Plans   97

Understanding the Nursing Process

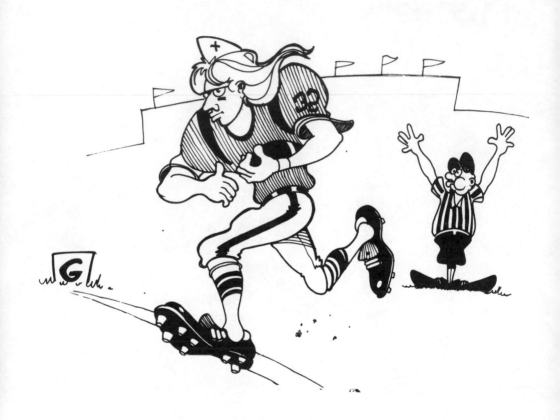

The Nursing Process

THE NURSE WHO SAVED FOOTBALL
(A Totally Untrue Story)

Long ago, before Howard Cosell had learned to talk, there existed a group of people with nothing to do on Sunday afternoons. One of them, John, was a very scholarly individual who had read about a game called football. He decided this game might give him and his friends something to do on those quiet Sundays. He told his friends all about the game and how it was played. Soon they all understood the game very well. They set up the field, erected goalposts, and bought a football. The next Sunday they were all set for some real action (on the field). They divided themselves into two teams and started to play. Now John, the scholarly individual, being the founder of the game, felt he should be the quarterback, since he weighed about 30 pounds less than everyone else and was no fool. Everyone agreed to this arrangement. John called his team into a huddle and said, "Let's get a goal!" so they lined up and started to play. After being sacked 47 times, John began to feel there was something wrong with his game. Football was definitely not a lot of fun for John that day. The next day at practice the team tried to figure out what went wrong. Some blamed John, some blamed the field, some wanted to quit and go back to being bored. One player, who worked as a nurse in a local hospital, said, "I think I have a suggestion. When I give nursing care I use the nursing process to develop a plan of care for my patients. I think our team needs to do the same thing and develop a GAME PLAN." So they did. They wrote a play book and coordinated their efforts to advance the ball. Of course, the next Sunday they creamed their opponents 70 to 3. And that's how the nursing process saved football.

THE NURSING PROCESS: WHAT IS IT?

The nursing process is a system of planning the delivery of nursing care, consisting of four steps:

1. **Assessment**
   What's the problem? How do I know it?
   Describe it.
   Is it animal, vegetable, or mineral?
2. **Planning**
   What are we going to do about it?
   What is the best strategy?
3. **Implementation**
   Move into action.
   Do it, to it!
4. **Evaluation**
   Did it work?
   How did it go?
   Did it fly, if it was supposed to?

An alternate breakdown of the nursing process is a five-step sequence which includes assessment, analysis, planning, implementation, and evaluation. A comparison of the four- and five-step format for the nursing process is shown in Table 1. This text uses the four-step breakdown of the nursing process but includes explanation of the analysis step in the chapters on assessment and planning.

Table 1   Comparison of the Four- and Five-Step Nursing Process Formats

Four-Step Format	Nursing Activities	Five-Step Format
1. Assessment	Collecting patient data Writing nursing diag- noses	1. Assessment
2. Planning	Setting priorities Writing patient care goals	2. Analysis
3. Implementation	Planning nursing actions Giving nursing care	3. Planning 4. Implementation
4. Evaluation	Evaluating goal achieve- ment Reassessing plan of care	5. Evaluation

The end product of this process is a written nursing care plan. While the above descriptions are an oversimplification, every nurse already has had much practice in using similar problem-solving techniques, even though the terms of the nursing process itself may be unfamiliar. Consider a high-school chemistry class. Students are asked to observe and examine the properties of different chemicals, and to perform a series of planned experiments utilizing those substances. The student then records and evaluates the results. Hopefully, the student, through the use of this scientific problem-solving process, has discovered the solution to the problem of how certain chemicals react. These steps are essentially the same as those utilized in the nursing process. More familiar is the case of the domestic engineer (uncommonly referred to as a father), who observes the chaos of his 7-year-old's bedroom. After giving the scene an eyeball ASSESSMENT, and palpating the bedcovers for any sign of life, he diagnoses the problem, "This room is an absolute mess!" He then sets forth a PLAN of action. He chooses a goal, "That child isn't going out to play until all his toys are put away." He recruits his son to IMPLEMENT the clean-up, and finally EVALUATES the results. These examples point out that a problem-solving process is important not only to the sciences but is also an integral activity of daily living. Similarly, the applied science of nursing utilizes a logical, systematic problem-solving process to deliver its services. This is called the nursing process. Patients' written care plans are based on application of the nursing process. These care plans serve as a guide for patient care.

WHY IS THE NURSING PROCESS IMPORTANT?

When used as a tool in nursing practice, the nursing process can help insure quality patient care. Without this systematic way of approaching patient care, omissions and duplications begin to occur. A nursing care plan helps to reduce these problems when it is used as a guide in providing care for a particular patient. Just as a physician formulates medical care plans in treating patients' diseases to insure consistent, responsible medical management, a nurse utilizes the nursing process to create care plans to insure consistent and responsible nursing management of patients' problems.

While the primary benefit of utilizing the nursing process is improved patient care, there are also definite advantages for the individual nurse who becomes skilled in the use of this tool. Consider the following advantages for the nurse (and the student):

1. **Graduation from an Accredited School of Nursing.** The National League for Nursing, which is the organization responsible for accrediting nursing programs, requires students to have a basic competency in the use of the nursing process upon graduation.*

2. **Confidence.** Care plans resulting from the nursing process let the student or the staff nurse know specifically what goals are important for the patient and how and when they might best be accomplished.

3. **Job Satisfaction.** Good care plans can save time, energy, and the frustration that is generated by trial-and-error nursing by staff members and students whose efforts remain uncoordinated. Coordinating a patient's nursing care through a care plan greatly increases the chances of achieving a successful resolution of health problems. The nurse and student should feel a real sense of accomplishment and professional pride when goals in a care plan are met.

4. **Professional Growth.** Care plans provide an opportunity to share knowledge and experience. Collaboration with colleagues in formulating a nursing care plan will add to an inexperienced nurse's clinical skills. Later, during the process of evaluation, the nurse or student receives the feedback necessary to decide how effective the nursing care plan was in dealing with the patient's problems. If the plan worked well, the nurse may use a similar approach in the future. If it failed, the nurse can explore possible reasons for the undesirable results with the patient, other staff, other students, an instructor, or a clinical nurse specialist.

5. **Aid in Staff Assignments.** Care plans assist charge nurses, team leaders, and nursing instructors in making the most appropriate patient assignments by showing the degree of complexity involved in an individual patient's care plan. Could an aide follow the care plan and provide good care, or is a professional nurse required? Could a student work with this patient, or is the plan of care beyond her knowledge and experience?

*NLN: *Competencies of the Associate Degree Nurse on Entry into Practice*; Pub. No. 23-1731; c. 1978; New York.

There are also advantages for the patient.

1. **Participation in Own Care.** If patients are able to help formulate their own care plans with the nurse, they gain a sense of their own ability to solve problems. When patients are active participants in their care, they are more likely to be committed to the goals in their care plans.

2. **Continuity of Care.** The frustration of repeating the same information to each nurse caring for them is greatly reduced. Worries, concerns, and problems need not be communicated to each nurse to ensure that they are handled the way patients want them to be handled. The care plan communicates this information.

3. **Improved Quality of Care.** Continuous evaluation and reassessment assures a level of care which will better meet changing individual needs. This evaluation is a key part of the nursing process and a patient's written care plan.

Giving nursing care without a care plan is like trying to cook a nameless entree without a recipe. To add to your troubles, you have to share the work for preparing this entree with three other cooks, all in the kitchen at different times. You can all cook, but a plan is needed to tell you what the entree is, how to prepare it, when to serve it, and how the three of you can coordinate your efforts to produce the best entree possible. Similarly, many nurses share in the care of a single patient throughout the 24-hour hospital day. Each nurse is capable of providing care, but a plan is needed to coordinate their efforts.

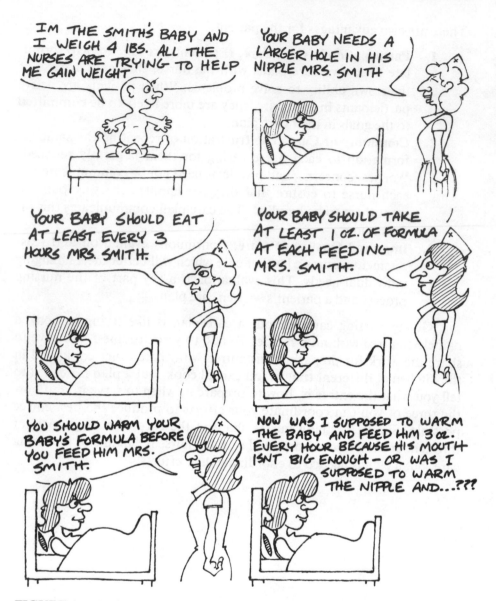

FIGURE 1. A plan is needed to coordinate the nurse's efforts.

WHAT DOES IT LOOK LIKE?

The use of the nursing process will result in a care plan describing the needs and care for each patient. You'll know you've discovered a nursing care plan when, while working in the clinical area, you find a nursing Kardex (by any other name a Kardex is still the same!) with a plan detailing the four elements of care: nursing diagnoses, goals, nursing actions, and evaluation.

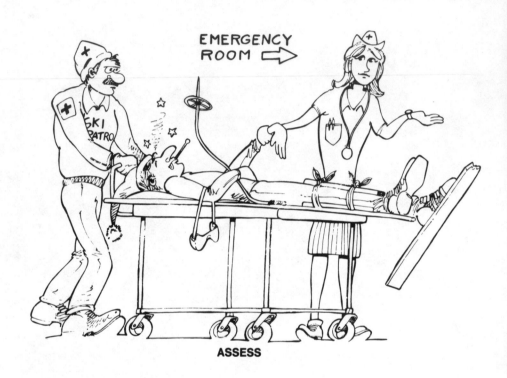

CHAPTER 1

Assessment

Assessment is the initial step in the nursing process and perhaps the most crucial, since the entire care plan is built upon the information gathered in this phase. The process of assessment consists of three separate interdependent activities: data collection, data organization, and formulating nursing diagnoses.

Assessment = Data Collection + Data Organization + Nursing Diagnoses

---

DATA COLLECTION

The nurse begins planning care for a particular patient through the activities of data collection. These activities begin at the time of patient admission and continue concurrently throughout each other phase of the nursing process. Observation, interviewing, and examination are three methods of collecting data. There are multiple sources of data available to the nurse. These sources include the patient as the primary source, the patient's chart, the family, and any other people giving care to the patient. Professional journals, reference texts, and clinical specialists are also important sources of data. Several sources should be used to assure completeness and reliability of the data. The patient is always a primary data source even if unable to communicate verbally. Observation and examination can be used to collect data from a non-verbal patient.

All nursing observations should result in objective data. Objective data are factual data which are observed by the nurse and could be noted by any other observer. The nurse describes the signs or behaviors observed without drawing conclusions or making interpretations. See Table 2 for examples of objective data.

The column of judgments and conclusions demonstrates the interpretations of one individual nurse. Consider that "neatly groomed" may mean different things to different individuals, whereas "hair combed, makeup applied" is concise and descriptive.

Contrasted with objective data are subjective data. Subjective data are information given verbally by the patient. Examples of this type of data are the following statements:

"I feel so nervous."
"My stomach is burning."
"I want to be alone now."

From the examples of subjective data listed above, each nurse could infer many different interpretations. For example, the nurse might guess that the patient was nervous because he fears that he has cancer. This interpretation is not justified on the basis of the patient's statement. The patient could be nervous for many different reasons. The task during the data collection phase is merely to observe, collect, and record data. Subjective data such as the examples in Table 3 are best recorded as direct quotes, thus providing the reader with the original information.

Table 2

Objective Data	Judgments and Conclusions
Hair combed, makeup applied	Neatly groomed
Drags right leg when walking	Walks with slight limp
Tremors of both hands	Patient very afraid
250 cc dark amber urine	Large amount urine
Patient in bed, covers over head, facing wall; no verbal response to questions	Patient depressed
Administered own 8 a.m. insulin	Understands self administration of insulin
Ate cereal, juice, toast, coffee	Good appetite

Table 3

Subjective Data	Judgments and Conclusions
"Get out of my room."	Hostile patient
"I know something is wrong with my baby."	Patient anxious
"This catheter is killing me."	Patient experiencing pain
"Where am I? How did I get here?"	Patient confused
"I'm afraid they will find cancer when they operate."	Patient worried about surgery

Observation

At the time of the first meeting with the patient, the nurse begins the observation phase of data collection which continues throughout the nurse-patient relationship. Every time the nurse is with the patient she should be gathering data through observation. Observation is a high

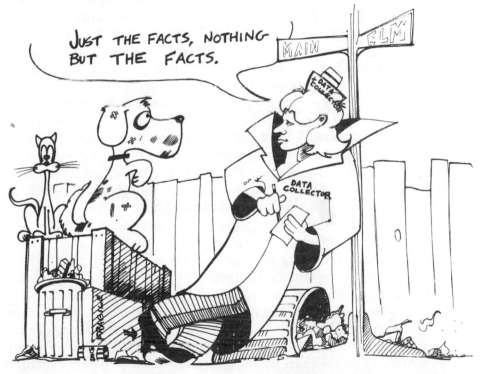

FIGURE 2. The nurse must record the observations without drawing conclusions.

level nursing skill which requires a great deal of practice. Consider the party game where each participant is required to view a tray holding many items. After a brief period of time the tray is removed and the participants are asked to list the items they can recall. Few people can successfully remember all of the items. The skills of observation and recall are difficult. The inexperienced student will find it hard to perform nursing tasks and simultaneously continue the observation process. Yet it is this ability to perform constant, ongoing observations that is essential to assessment. For example, a nursing student giving a first backrub is concentrating so hard on the task that she is unable to make observations. As students gain skill in giving physical care, they can shift their attention to the total patient and begin to collect data through observation.

Interview

Just as the observation phase of data collection is ongoing, the nursing interview is also continuous during the nurse-patient relationship. Interviewing can be done both formally and informally. A formal interview consists of purposeful communication during which the nurse takes the nursing history of the patient. Unlike the medical history which has the disease process as its primary focus, the nursing history considers the patient's perception of his illness and his response to it. The purpose of this interview is to help the nurse obtain information which will help in planning nursing care for the patient. This purpose should be clearly and directly communicated to the patient at the beginning of the interview. Due to the comprehensive nature of the nursing history some aspects of the medical history may be included, though the nurse will attempt to eliminate duplication of data. Many hospital admission formats include a nursing history page which is retained as a part of the patient's permanent record.

Frequently, beginning nursing students have difficulty eliciting a nursing history, complaining that they feel they are prying into personal matters. Students may be assured that the patient has the right to refuse to discuss any topic and that this right must be respected. When patients do reveal personal data, they can be further assured of the confidentiality of the nurse-patient relationship. Such data will remain within the context of the professional relationship and will be used only in matters related to providing patient care. The formal nursing interview is not intended to be a treatment in and of itself, but is rather an organized format for data collection. Frequently, however, the patient has a need to express feelings and the nursing interview provides the opportunity and the uninterrupted attention of the nurse. This is often therapeutic for the patient.

The informal aspect of the nursing interview is the conversation between the nurse and patient during the course of giving nursing care. The close relationship developed while the nurse is giving physical care frequently enables the patient to express feelings and problems. The nurse who can skillfully give physical care is then free to simultaneously focus attention on what the patient is saying.

Examination

The final activity of data collection is examination. Before beginning the physical process of examination, the nurse must establish a relationship with the patient. The nurse must also precede the examination by an introduction and identification of herself. She then provides an explanation of her examination and requests the patient's permission to proceed. Provision for the patient's privacy (close both door and curtains, please!) must be made. Then the nurse may examine the patient, completing such observations as TPR (temperature, pulse, respiration), BP (blood pressure), chest and heart sounds, and skin problems, paying particular attention to any physical complaints the patient may have mentioned. In obtaining this data, the nurse may use a cephalo-caudal approach (head to toe), or perhaps a body systems approach to examination (i.e., respiratory, digestive, cardiovascular, etc.). While it is necessary to establish a relationship with the patient prior to examination, the examination itself can also be a tool for showing concern and enhancing a relationship. The nurse who stops to palpate the abdomen and listen to bowel sounds when the patient complains of pain, shows concern for the patient and establishes herself as a credible clinician. The observations the nurse makes during an examination should be recorded as objective data: 3-inch scar, left lower quadrant; temperature 98°F; BP 110/70; lungs sounds normal and clear.

During the assessment phase the nurse has the potential to collect volumes of data about a client. Throughout the process it is important to consider the significance of the data to the task at hand which is identifying problems and planning nursing intervention. As the student practices data collection, skill must be used in selecting data and eliciting relevant data.

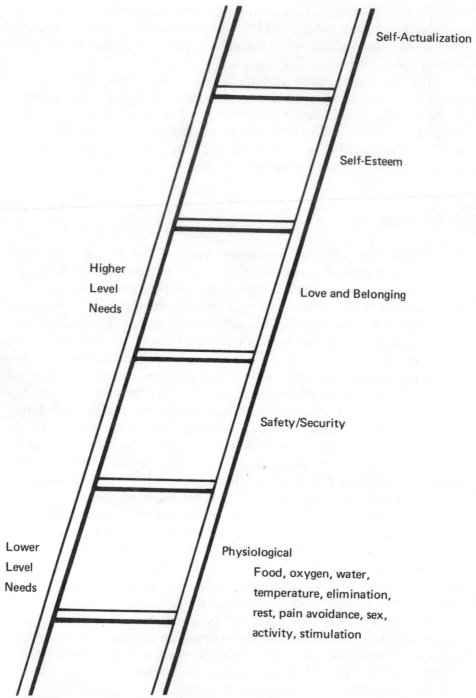

Self-Actualization

Self-Esteem

Higher
Level
Needs

Love and Belonging

Safety/Security

Lower
Level
Needs

Physiological
   Food, oxygen, water,
   temperature, elimination,
   rest, pain avoidance, sex,
   activity, stimulation

FIGURE 3.   Maslow's hierarchy of human needs.

DATA ORGANIZATION

"So now that I've got all this data, what do I do with it?"
"Organize it to make it useful!"

There are many ways of organizing data, but each nurse should be guided by pragmatism, that is, use what works best for you! One way of viewing data is based on work of psychologist Abraham Maslow. He postulated that all human beings have common basic needs which can be arranged in the following hierarchical order (see Table 4). Maslow further theorized that basic physical needs must be met to some degree before higher level needs can be met.

The basic physical needs such as food, fluid, and oxygen are considered survival needs and must be met, or at least partially met, if life is to continue. They are the lowest level of needs and usually are satisfied before higher level needs. Higher level needs begin with safety/security needs and continue through self-actualization needs.

Using Maslow's theory, consider the following data and the way they are organized.

1. **Physiological needs**
   —temperature 103°F.
   —respirations 36 per minute.
   —liquid stool four times in one hour.
   —complains of sharp continuous pain in right lower quadrant.
2. **Safety/security needs**
   —sleeps with night light.
   —mother says 4-year-old Billy is afraid of dark.
   —"I want my mama!"

Table 4

1. Physiological needs—needs which must be met for survival
2. Safety and security needs—things which make the person feel safe and comfortable
3. Love and belonging needs—the need to give and receive love and affection
4. Esteem needs—things that make a person feel good about himself; pride in one's ability and accomplishments
5. Self-actualization needs—the need to continue to grow and change; working toward future goals

3. **Love and belonging**
   —mother and father with Billy.
   —has an infant brother at home.
4. **Self-esteem**
   —"I can dress myself."
   —"I hate bedpans. Only babies go in bed."
   —"I can say the alphabet and count to 20."
5. **Self-actualization**
   —"When I can ride my bike real good, my Mom will take the
   training wheels off."
   —"I'm getting ready for kindergarten."

The data recorded within each category may indicate the current
status of need satisfaction, alterations in meeting the need, or perhaps
interferences in meeting the need. By collecting data in each of these
need categories, the nurse develops a format for systematically considering the total patient rather than viewing an illness or a symptom. Comprehensive nursing care results from a consideration of the total patient.

In addition to classifying data using the need levels of Maslow,
some consideration of the individual's level of growth and development
is necessary. Each chronological age has corresponding developmental
tasks, both physical and psychosocial. A developmental task may be
thought of as a job, a hurdle, a challenge, or an accomplishment relative to a particular chronological age span. Illness may interfere with
completion of developmental tasks appropriate to an age span or with
progression to the next developmental level. During illness an individual
may even regress to an earlier level of development. For example, the 3-
year-old who has been toilet trained for 6 months may begin bed wetting
again during hospitalization. The adolescent who has been menstruat-
ing for 6 months may cease to menstruate during lengthy confinement
in a body cast. Other individuals may appear to arrest at a developmental level during the stress of illness and hospitalization. For example, an
infant may fail to begin to crawl and stand during illness. The infant
may remain at the developmental level achieved prior to hospitalization
and show very little new learning until the stress of hospitalization and
illness is reduced. Thus it is important for the nurse to assess developmental levels and the tasks associated with each level so she can recognize and understand variations from normal age-related development in
patients. By recognizing that a child is regressing to an earlier level or is
failing to keep up with his peers' development, the nurse may be able to

work with the parents and other hospital staff to reduce the damaging influence that hospitalization may have on a child's development. The nurse who has a knowledge of developmental levels and the associated tasks will be able to further individualize patient care. For example, adolescent developmental tasks focus on self-identity. While caring for adolescents, the nurse could choose a nonauthoritative approach which would allow the patient the maximum amount of choice in his care. Similarly, a school-age child's developmental level focuses on independence and project completion. Nursing care that encourages the child to do as much as he can for himself will promote developmental growth. Table 5 is a very brief summary of developmental tasks and the corresponding age spans.

Table 5

Major Developmental Tasks

1. Infancy—1 year
   —developing a sense of trust and belonging from relationship with mother and father
   —differentiating self from environment
   —learning to eat solid foods, to walk, to explore, to communicate
2. Toddler—1–3 years
   —developing will power, independence
   —learning to feed self, to run, communicate verbally, control elimination
   —exploring environment
3. Preschool—3–6 years
   —developing sexual identity
   —developing a sense of initiative
   —working on autonomy, dressing self, washing
   —developing sense of time, space, distance
   —developing imagination
   —playing cooperatively
4. School Age—6–puberty
   —developing a sense of industry; planning and working on projects
   —learning the skills for survival in the child's culture
   —developing modesty
   —learning to read, to calculate, to control emotions
   —developing neuromuscular coordination
5. Adolescent—12–18 years
   —developing physical maturity
   —developing autonomy from home and family
   —developing self-identity
   —coping with body image
   —identifying with peer group

Table 5 (cont.)

6. Early Adult—18–40 years
    —forming lasting relationships; marriage, career choice; caring for others
    —parenting role, to nurture and guide the next generation
    —responsibilities greatly increased
    —adjusting to aging parents
7. Middle Adult—40–65 years
    —adjusting to decreased metabolism, altered hormone levels, decreased
      visual acuity and hearing
    —adjusting to independence of children and dependence of aged parents
    —coping with physical and emotional changes of aging
    —establishing financial security
8. Senior Adult—65 years to death
    —coping with increased incidence of chronic disease
    —forming second and third generation relationships
    —facing own death and adjusting to death of spouse and friends
    —altering expressions of sexuality
    —developing goals for meaningful life
    —maintaining health

The case study method will be used throughout this book to illustrate the steps of the nursing process. The same case study of Mrs. Smith will be found in each chapter, ending in a nursing care plan for a hospital Kardex. The worksheet (Figure 4) illustrates data collection and organization for Mrs. Smith.

Note the placement and classification of data according to Maslow and growth and development on the nursing care plan worksheet which follows. It is not important that this exact format for writing nursing care plans be used. However, a consistent method for writing the plan provides a framework for a student or nurse who is trying to learn to use the nursing process. Do not be alarmed at the length of the example of the written care plan. This was done for the purpose of clarifying the process for the beginner. A final chapter will show an abbreviated format for use in the hospital. Similarly, as the nurse gains skill in using the nursing process, many of the steps may be done without writing them. In complex cases, the nurse may still choose to write the steps as an aid to planning care.

NURSING CARE PLAN WORKSHEET   CASE STUDY: Mrs. Smith

Data

1. 45-year-old white female.
2. Mother of 13- and 17-year-old sons.
3. Married.
4. 11/6 Admitted 11:30 p.m. via emergency room complaining of vomiting, feeling hot, flushed, dry skin, abdominal pain.
5. Blood sugar 240 mg per ml on admission, urine 4 + glucose.
6. Prior to admission shared large pizza and coke with husband.
7. Voiding q.2h 250–300 cc urine.
8. 11/9 Diagnosis of diabetes mellitus.
9. Height 5'4", weight 150 lb
10. "I'm always hungry but lately I've lost 10 lb without even trying. I've never been able to diet successfully."
11. "I drink coffee and tea constantly throughout the day. I always have a cup going."
12. 11/7 Intake 3000 cc, output 2800 cc.
13. Activity: bridge club twice a week, flower gardening, housework.
14. 11/8 Fasting blood sugar: 180 mg per 100 ml.
15. "I had a bad cold last week. I was just beginning to feel better."
16. "Lately I've been so cranky. I argue with the boys over nothing."
17. "The boys are really nice children. I work hard at being their mother and I'm proud of them."
18. "I'm almost never sick and now to have to take medicine daily,

Data Organization

Maslow's Needs:

1. Physical
   1, 4, 5, 6, 7, 8, 9, 10, 11, 12, 14, 15, 22
2. Safety/security
   8, 24, 25
3. Love and belonging
   2, 3, 13, 16, 19, 20, 23
4. Self-esteem
   10, 13, 18, 21, 24, 25
5. Self-actualization
   17
6. Growth and development
   1, 2, 3, 17

NURSING CARE PLAN WORKSHEET (Cont.)

     to be on a special diet, well . . .
     that's just not me.''

19. ''I can't make my family suffer
     just because I'm on a diabetic
     diet.''

20. ''Meal time is a special time in
     our day. We're all together
     and we really enjoy the meal.
     Now. . . .''

21. ''I love to cook, especially the
     rich chocolate desserts we all
     love. The boys just inhale des-
     serts and cookies.''

22. ''I'm not a breakfast person—
     just can't face food at that
     hour.''

23. ''And what about bridge club?
     We always munch. That's
     part of the fun. If I can't do
     that. . . .''

24. ''Am I going to go blind?''

25. ''Diabetics often have to have
     feet amputated, don't they?''

FIGURE 4.   Sample nursing care plan worksheet showing data collected and organized according to Maslow's hierarchy of needs.

NURSING DIAGNOSIS

The final step in the assessment process is the formulation of nursing diagnoses. In a five-step nursing process format, interpretation of data and determination of nursing diagnoses are part of the analysis step, as are priority setting and selection of patient care goals. These activities are discussed in Chapter 2 of this text as part of the planning step.

NURSING DIAGNOSIS:

a statement of a present or potential patient problem that requires nursing intervention in order to be resolved or lessened.

The nursing diagnosis must be a problem. If it is not a problem, no nursing diagnosis need be made. Consider the bowel function status of a patient restricted to bed rest. If the patient has a soft, formed stool without exertion every 2 to 3 days, elimination is not a problem and no nursing diagnosis need be made. However, the nurse must also consider who defines a problem. If the patient considers it abnormal not to have a daily bowel movement and continues to express anxiety related to this, a problem does exist as defined by the patient. The nurse may understand that physiologically no problem exists, but that the patient could benefit from teaching regarding normal body function. Nursing care may then focus on teaching as an intervention tool to reduce anxiety.

As defined here, the problem expressed in the nursing diagnosis may be either present or potential. A present nursing diagnosis refers to a situation existing in the here and now. A patient on a general diet with a good appetite has not had a bowel movement for 4 days, complains of low abdominal pain, and is unable to pass stool. This patient is constipated and requires assistance. This is a current problem for the patient.

A potential problem refers to a situation which may cause difficulty in the future. By identifying the potential problem, the nurse may be able to prevent the problem or lessen its consequences. If a patient is on absolute bed rest while in a full leg cast, the patient is at risk for developing bedsores (decubitus ulcers) due to inactivity and decreased circulation. Understanding the physiological effects of bed rest, the nurse may take action to prevent bed sores. In this case, the problem is a potential one which requires preventive nursing intervention. The potential nursing diagnosis is made based on the nurse's past experience in similar situations and on an understanding of pathophysiology. The problem would predictably occur without nursing intervention.

In still other situations, the nurse may wish to formulate a tentative nursing diagnosis. This type of nursing diagnosis may be made when the nurse has insufficient data from an individual patient to support a firm nursing diagnosis. This may be compared to the physician who lists several "rule out" medical diagnoses in a patient's admission assessment. By considering such a tentative nursing diagnosis, the nurse assures continued collection of relevant data. With an increased data base, the nurse may be able to firmly establish the tentative nursing diagnosis as valid or to eliminate the tentative nursing diagnosis as invalid for this particular patient. For example:

An adolescent has arrived in the emergency room to receive stitches for a scalp laceration. Treatment requires that a large portion of her head be shaved. The nurse considers a tentative nursing diagnosis of decreased self-esteem related to loss of hair. The nurse bases this diagnosis on her knowledge of growth and development, since most adolescents are very concerned about their physical appearance. Note, however, that this diagnosis is not supported by data from this individual patient. This diagnosis is based on inference at this point and thus is tentative. The nurse seeks to gather more data to support her diagnosis. The nurse uses interviewing skills in collecting more data as she asks the patient, "A lot of girls might be very upset about having their hair cut. How do you feel about this?" The patient replies, "No problem, I wear lots of wigs." The nurse may then eliminate that tentative diagnosis.

The following formula will result in a clear concise statement of a nursing diagnosis.

Nursing Diagnosis = Patient Problem + Cause if Known

Nothing, repeat, nothing else, belongs in the nursing diagnosis. Keep it clean! When beginning it may be helpful to state a nursing diagnosis and then identify the data upon which that nursing diagnosis is based. This helps to assure that a nursing diagnosis is accurate and is based upon facts. A nursing diagnosis is not an inference. If you are unable to identify the data upon which a nursing diagnosis is based, there are two alternatives. You may go back and collect more data, or you may write a tentative nursing diagnosis to assure the continuance of data collection. Both alternatives stress the necessity of supporting the nursing diagnosis by using data. The following suggestions may also guide you in formulating nursing diagnoses:

1. Keep nursing diagnoses brief.
2. Keep nursing diagnoses specific.
3. Each nursing diagnosis relates to one patient problem.
4. Each nursing diagnosis must be based on patient data.

The following examples combine these elements to form nursing diagnoses.

Problem	+	Cause if Known
1. Pain		associated with surgical incision
2. Poor vision		related to bilateral cataracts
3. Difficulty breathing		associated with congestive heart failure
4. Boredom		related to isolation procedure
5. Moderate anxiety		related to unknown medical diagnosis
6. Diarrhea		related to viral influenza
7. Prone to injury		related to organic brain syndrome
8. Prone to impaired wound healing		related to malnourished status

A nursing diagnosis is not synonymous with a medical diagnosis. The following comparison may help to clarify what constitutes a nursing diagnosis.

A Nursing Diagnosis	
Is	*Is Not*
A statement of a patient problem	A medical diagnosis
Actual or potential	A nursing action
Within the scope of nursing intervention	A physician's order
Suggestive of nursing intervention	A therapeutic treatment

Frequently a medical diagnosis may suggest nursing diagnoses.

Medical Diagnosis	*Nursing Diagnosis*
Peptic ulcer	Pain related to peptic ulcer
Myocardial infarction	Anxiety related to myocardial infarction
Cerebral vascular accident	Altered ability to perform activities of daily living (ADL) related to cerebrovascular accident (CVA; stroke)
Chronic ulcerative colitis	Alteration in bowel elimination
Acute myelogenous leukemia	Prone to infection related to AML
Senile bilateral cataract	Prone to injury related to poor vision
Cancer of breast	Alteration of body image related to mastectomy

Table 6 lists nursing diagnoses which are currently acceptable and others to be developed by the Clearinghouse, National Group for Classification of Nursing Diagnosis. These problem statements are intended to provide an initial standardized listing of nursing diagnosis. The listing is not yet complete, however, and the problem you identify may not necessarily be included. Do not hesitate to add your problem statements to the listing.

PRACTICE EXERCISE

Pick out the correctly written nursing diagnoses. Identify what is wrong with the incorrectly written nursing diagnoses. The answers are on the following pages.

1. Loss of appetite related to chemotherapy
2. Range-of-motion (ROM) exercises associated with stroke
3. Cancer of breast related to primary site
4. Refusing wound irrigation related to pain of procedure
5. Altered body image related to amputation of right foot
6. Prone to altered sexual identity and sexual behavior in relating to husband and friends related to breast cancer
7. Intermittent positive pressure breathing (IPPB) exercises q.i.d. to increase lung expansion
8. Pain and fear related to surgical procedure
9. Severe itching related to fungal infection
10. Delayed wound healing related to poor nutritional intake
11. Inability to move right side associated with right-side paralysis
12. Respiratory distress at birth
13. Disoriented to time and place related to confused state
14. Difficulty communicating related to native Spanish language
15. Anxiety related to nervous tension
16. Ambulate progressively
17. Prone to infection related to second degree burn
18. Patient is upset and worried
19. Difficulty walking associated with prolonged bed rest
20. Thrombophlebitis related to prolonged bed rest

Table 6

Nursing Diagnoses

Accepted

Airway clearance, ineffective

Bowel elimination, alterations in:
Constipation

Bowel elimination, alterations in:
Diarrhea

Bowel elimination, alterations in:
Incontinence

Breathing patterns, ineffective

Cardiac output, alterations in: Decreased

Comfort, alterations in: Pain

Communication, impaired verbal

Coping, ineffective individual

Coping, ineffective family: Compromised

Coping ineffective family: Disabling

Coping, family: Potential for
growth

Diversional activity, deficit

Fear, (specify)

Fluid volume deficit, actual

Fluid volume deficit, potential

Gas exchange, impaired

Grieving, anticipatory

Grieving, dysfunctional

Home maintenance management,
impaired

Injury, potential for

Knowledge deficit (specify)

Mobility, impaired physical

Noncompliance (specify)

Nutrition, alterations in: Less than
body requirements

Nutrition, alterations in: More than
body requirements

Nutrition, alterations in: Potential
for more than body requirements

Parenting, alterations in: Actual

Parenting, alterations in: Potential

Rape-trauma syndrome

Self-care deficit (specify level):
Feeding, bathing/hygiene, dressing/grooming, toileting

Self-concept, disturbance in

Sensory perceptual alterations

Sexual dysfunction

Skin integrity, impairment of: Actual

Skin integrity, impairment of: Potential

Sleep pattern disturbance

Spiritual distress (distress of the human spirit)

Thought processes, alterations in

Tissue perfusion, alterations in

Urinary elimination, alterations in
patterns

Violence, potential for

New Diagnosis Accepted for Clinical Testing, April 1982, Fifth National Conference On Classification of Nursing Diagnosis

Activity intolerance

Anxiety

Family processes, alteration in

Fluid volume, alteration in: Excess

Health maintenance alteration

Oral mucus membrane, alterations
in

Powerlessness

Social isolation

Reprinted with permission of the National Group for the Classification of Nursing Diagnosis, St. Louis, Missouri.

ANSWERS TO EXERCISE ON NURSING DIAGNOSIS

EVALUATION	RATIONALE
1. Correct	Problem = loss of appetite Cause = chemotherapy
2. Incorrect	ROM exercise is a nursing action
3. Incorrect	This is a medical diagnosis
4. Incorrect	This is a nursing problem– not a patient problem
5. Correct	Problem = altered body image Cause = amputation of right foot
6. Incorrect	Vague and nonspecific Multiple problems Too long
7. Incorrect	This is medical treatment
8. Incorrect	Two separate problems
9. Correct	Problem = severe itching Cause = fungal infection
10. Correct	Problem = delayed wound healing Cause = poor nutritional intake
11. Incorrect	Problem and cause are the same
12. Correct	Problem = Respiratory distress Cause = Unknown
13. Incorrect	Problem and cause are same
14. Correct	Problem = Difficulty communicating Cause = Native Spanish speaker
15. Incorrect	Problem and cause are same
16. Incorrect	This is physician's order
17. Correct	Problem = Prone to infection Cause = Second degree burn
18. Incorrect	Vague and nonspecific

ANSWERS TO EXERCISE ON NURSING DIAGNOSIS (Cont.)

EVALUATION	RATIONALE
19. Correct	Problem = Difficulty walking Cause = Prolonged bed rest
20. Incorrect	Thrombophlebitis is a medical diagnosis

The following nursing diagnoses are based on data from the case study of Mrs. Smith. The nursing process will be used to plan nursing care to resolve the five problems in the chapters to follow.

Nursing Diagnosis   CASE STUDY: Mrs. Smith

		Problem	Plus	Cause	Data[a]
Present	{	1. Inadequate information	related to	diabetes mellitus	16, 18, 19, 23, 24, 25
		2. Fear	related to	possible complications of diabetes mellitus	24, 25
		3. Altered body image	related to	diagnosis of diabetes mellitus	10, 18, 22, 23, 24
		4. Prone to hyperglycemia	related to	family/personal eating habits	5, 6, 8, 10, 14, 19, 20, 21, 22, 23
Potential	{	5. Prone to skin infections	related to	diabetes mellitus	5, 8, 9

[a] Numbers listed under Data refer to original data base pp. 19–20.

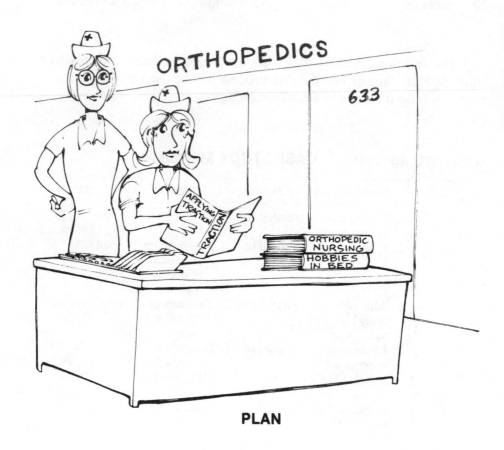

PLAN

CHAPTER 2

PLANNING

Now that you have gathered your patient's data, organized the data, and formulated some nursing diagnoses, you are ready to begin the planning phase of the nursing process. This is the time to develop a plan of care, and to determine what approach you are going to use to help solve, lessen, or minimize the effect of your patient's problems. In the planning phase, the nurse applies the skills of problem solving and decision making to a particular patient's identified problems. There are three steps in the planning phase: setting priorities, writing goals, and planning nursing actions.

Planning = Setting Priorities + Writing Goals + Planning Nursing Actions

---

SETTING PRIORITIES

Priority setting is the step during which the nurse and the patient determine the order in which the patient's problems should be approached. Which nursing diagnosis poses the greatest threat to the patient's well-being? The nursing diagnosis given the highest priority will be designated as problem number one and treated first. Subsequent problems are then numbered two, three, four, etc. Setting priorities serves the purpose of ordering the delivery of nursing care so more important problems are considered before lesser problems. Priority setting does not mean that one problem must be totally resolved before another problem can be considered. Problems can frequently be approached simultaneously. How does the nurse decide which problem should be given the highest priority? These guidelines may help you in selecting the nursing diagnosis which should be ranked first.

1. Maslow's hierarchy of basic needs can guide your selection of a priority need. Lower needs must usually be met before an individual can focus on higher needs. For example:

    Relieve a patient's pain (physiological need) before you encourage him to do morning hygiene (self-esteem need). Encourage a new mother to talk about her experience in labor (self-esteem need) before expecting her to take on the new role of mothering with great involvement (self-actualization need). Stabilize bleeding and insure adequate oxygenation in an emergency room accident victim before assessing elimination status: Both of these are basic physiological needs but oxygenation is usually the highest priority need; bleeding is considered a threat to tissue oxygen needs.

    Consider how difficult it is for you to read and absorb the material in this book (self-actualization need) if you have had too little sleep (physiological need). Basic survival needs will usually take priority over higher level needs if the survival needs are not being satisfied. This is the case when a patient is in obvious physical distress due to the unmet need. If the survival needs are being partially met and actual physical distress is minimal, a higher level need may take priority or at least have the same priority as a lower level need. For example, an auto accident victim can be in considerable distress with multiple physical needs unmet, yet the priority need may be to ascertain the whereabouts and injuries of the other family members in the car when it crashed. This unmet higher level need can have a negative effect on satisfaction of this patient's physical needs if it is not given appropriate attention.

2. Meet the needs the patient feels are most important if this order does not interfere with medical treatment. A patient's need for undisturbed rest cannot take precedence over a medical treatment which requires the observation of blood pressure and pulse every hour following a car accident. If there are no contraindications, offer patients the opportunity to set their own priorities. This serves two purposes. First, this approach involves patients in planning their own care. Perhaps the nurse has overlooked a major problem which is consuming the patient's time and energy. Unless this problem is considered first,

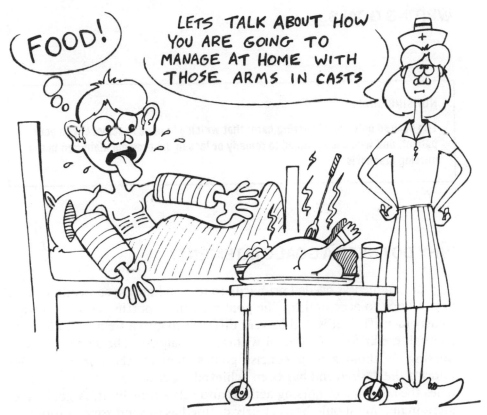

FIGURE 5. Priority setting.

the nurse may be able to achieve only a limited success in other areas because the patient is still worrying about the overlooked problem. Second, cooperation between the nurse and the patient is enhanced when priority setting is done together.

3. Consider the potential effect of future problems when setting priorities. For example:

A new mother may ask to be left alone with her husband and baby to get acquainted. The potential problem of a postpartum hemorrhage would require continuous observation after delivery, since this is potentially life threatening. Thus the patient's request to be left alone cannot be safely met.

A bedridden patient may need to start on a routine of frequent turning and positioning to prevent bed sores and contractures, even though the patient may not see this as important. Prevention of the potential complications of prolonged bedrest is a high priority need.

WRITING GOALS

NURSING GOAL:

The desired outcome of nursing care; that which you hope to achieve with your patient, and which is designed to remedy or lessen the problem identified in the nursing diagnosis.

WHY DO I NEED A GOAL STATEMENT?

A goal statement is needed primarily to let you know specifically what it is you hope to accomplish. The goal area in a sporting event is always clearly identified. It would be very difficult to give a field goal kicker in football credit for a field goal without a goalpost. The same is true in nursing. Without a clear concise goal statement, the nurse does not know if the desired end has been achieved. A clear goal statement identifies the outcome of nursing actions and sets a time limit. A goal statement in nursing should be as clearly defined as the end zone in football. Any nurse observing the patient after reading the nursing goal should be able to decide if the goal was reached.

Some goals in nursing care are similar to learning objectives for a course of study. A nursing goal may actually be a learning objective if the nursing diagnosis relates to a lack of patient knowledge or skill. The goal, like a learning objective in education, is written to identify the learning or improved performance that the nurse hopes will occur, following patient teaching. All goals are not learning objectives. Only those goals related to improving a patient's understanding, knowledge base, or skill in an area would qualify as learning goals or learning objectives.

There are two broad categories of goals: short-term goals and long-term goals. Short-term goals are outcomes which can be met fairly quickly, in a matter of hours or days. Short-term goals are especially appropriate to acute care settings or emergency situations where patients are unstable and long-term outcomes are uncertain. For example:

SHORT-TERM GOALS

1. Patient will verbalize a decrease in pain within 45 minutes of administration of pain medication.
2. Return of bowel sounds or passing flatus, 24 hours post-op.
3. Respiratory rate within normal range in 2 hours.
4. Intake of 2000 cc for 24 hours.
5. Fetal heart rate remains normal during labor and delivery.

A series of short-term goals can be written to gradually advance a patient toward a long-term goal. A long-term goal of losing 100 pounds in one year could be met by the following sequence of short-term goals:

Progressive Short-Term Goals

1. "I will weigh 210 pounds by February 7."
2. "I will weigh 208 pounds by February 14."
3. "I will weigh 206 pounds by February 21."

A series of short-term goals which a person can realistically accomplish in a stated time period is much more rewarding than striving for one long-term goal. The repeated reinforcement a person receives from meeting short-term goals can keep an individual motivated to reach a long-term goal.

LONG-TERM GOALS

Long-term goals are outcomes which cover a longer time span. There are two types of long-term goals. The first type covers an extended period of time and requires continuous nursing actions dealing *directly* with that goal for its accomplishment. For example, a patient prone to skin breakdown related to the effects of prolonged bedrest requires continuous nursing actions during the entire hospital stay to prevent skin breakdown. A long-term goal might state "Prevention of skin breakdown while on bedrest." The nursing actions of turning, repositioning, using an alternating pressure air mattress, and massaging the patient deal directly with the achievement of this long-term goal. The second type of long-term goal is best met by a progression of short-term goals.

Each progressive short-term goal requires a series of nursing actions for its accomplishment. This second type of long-term goal does not require a set of direct nursing actions, since the nursing actions accompany the progressive short-term goals. For example:

1. "I will finish reading this book before final exams," might be a long-term goal for a student in nursing. This student might accomplish the long-term goal by progressive short-term goals of reading one chapter each week.
2. "Patient will demonstrate full use of broken arm within 6 months." This patient might accomplish the long-term goal by progressively increasing the amount and range of muscle/joint exercises.
3. "Performance of self care activities within 3 months of cerebral vascular accident (stroke)." Progressive short-term goals might focus on accomplishment of one self care activity a week until the patient was able to perform the activity independently.
    Week of 10/10: Feeding self by end of week.
    Week of 10/17: Brushing teeth by end of week.
    Week of 10/24: Performs personal hygiene by end of week.
    Week of 10/31: Meets own mobility needs by end of week.

The following suggestions may be helpful as you begin to write goal statements for your nursing diagnoses.

1. **The goal statement should be a patient behavior which demonstrates reduction or alleviation of the problem identified in the nursing diagnosis.** Start with the nursing diagnosis. What is the problem? If the nursing diagnosis is "Pain due to broken right arm," the goal should demonstrate alleviation or lessening of the pain. If the nursing diagnosis is "Fear of being unable to breast-feed baby due to previous failure with first child," the goal should involve alleviating or lessening her fear of failing at breast-feeding. If the nursing diagnosis is "Alterations in bowel elimination," the goal should deal with bowel elimination patterns and reestablishing normal function, if possible.
2. **The goal should be realistic for the patient's capabilities in the time span you designate in your goal.** A goal for a preterm baby, weighing 4 pounds, that stated "Baby will weigh 8 pounds at the end of 1 week," would be unrealistic for this newborn. But if the goal stated "Baby will weigh 4½ pounds

in 7 days," the capabilities of the patient have been considered and make the goal more realistic and more likely to be achieved. Experience, professional literature, references, and advice from other more experienced nurses will help the student learn what is realistic for patients with particular problems.

3. **The goal should be realistic for the nurse's level of skill and experience.** If the nursing diagnosis is dealing with a problem beyond the nurse's role, the best course of action is to refer the problem to the appropriate professional. A patient with a nursing diagnosis of "Malnutrition related to refusal to eat hospital food," should be referred to a dietician. A patient with a nursing diagnosis of "Inability to speak related to recent stroke," should be referred to a speech therapist when the patient's condition is sufficiently stable.

4. **The goal should be congruent with and supportive of other therapies.** This means that nursing goals for the patient should not contradict or interfere with the work of other professionals caring for the patient. If the nursing diagnosis is "Muscle weakness due to bedrest" and the physician has ordered bedrest for 2 more weeks, a nursing goal involving getting the patient out of bed would contradict the medical order and be inappropriate.

5. **Whenever possible the goal should be important and valued by the patient, the nurses and the physician.** If the goals are important to the patients, they will be more motivated to reach a goal. If nurses value the goal, they will be more likely to carry out the suggested plan of care. The physician's understanding and support of nursing goals will help to assure congruence with medical treatment. The goals also serve as a communication tool which keeps health team members informed of the patient's progress.

6. **When you start to write goals, start with short-term goals.** As a beginning nursing student, you are not with the same patient for long periods of time. You may only care for the patient for 1 or 2 days. If you write a short-term goal involving the length of time you plan to be with the patient, you will be able to give the needed nursing care and evaluate the results yourself. By evaluating if your goal was met before you leave the patient, you will gain skill in writing realistic goals and in giving nursing care to meet those goals.

General Guidelines to Goal Writing

1. Write goals in observable or measurable terms whenever possible. Try to avoid words such as good, normal, adequate, and improved. These words mean different things to different people and tend to make the goal unclear. There may be disagreement as to whether the goal was achieved if words requiring a judgment are used in the goal statement.

Observable Goal	Vague Goal
The patient will walk the length of the hall unassisted by 2/5.	Increased ambulation or Adequate leg strength
Patient will gain 1/4 lb each week until discharged.	Increased intake or Good nutrition or Promote weight gain

2. Write goals in terms of patient outcomes, not nursing actions.

Patient Outcomes	Nursing Actions
The patient will void by 6 p.m.	I will offer the patient the urinal every 2 hours.
The patient will bathe her baby before she is discharged.	I will show the patient a baby bath before she is discharged.
The patient's temperature will be up to 98 °F within 1 hour.	I will put warm blankets and a heating pad on the patient and recheck his temperature in 1 hour.

3. Keep the goal short.
4. Make the goal specific.
5. Each goal is derived from only one nursing diagnosis.
6. Designate a specific time for achievement of each goal. Write either the date the goal was written or the date for evaluation.

If the goal is to be achieved within a matter of hours, times may be used rather than dates.

FORMULA FOR WRITING A GOAL

Subject + Verb + Criteria of Performance + Conditions = Goal
(if needed)   Statement

SUBJECT = the patient or any part of the patient; a noun. The subject may be omitted when writing a goal in a care plan. It is assumed unless otherwise indicated.
—the patient's pulse
—the patient's urinary output
—the patient's ulcer
—the patient
VERB = the action that the subject (the patient) will perform
CRITERIA OF ACCEPTABLE PERFORMANCE = the level at which the patient will perform a certain behavior. How well? How long? How far? How much?
    The criteria of acceptable performance contains a designated time or date for achievement of the behavior.
—by the time of discharge
—at the end of this shift
—by 6/4
—by 2 p.m. today
CONDITION = the circumstances, if important, under which the behavior will be performed. All goals will not have a condition. If the condition is important, put it in the goal statement; if it is not important, leave it out.
—with the help of a walker
—with the use of a wheelchair
—with the help of the family
—with the use of medications

The following examples combine these elements to form goal statements.

Subject	+ Verb	+ Criteria	+ Condition (if relevant)
The patient	will void	at least 100 cc by 6 p.m. tonight.	
PO$_2$	will be	within the normal range by 10 p.m.	
The patient	will walk	up and down stairs by the time of discharge	with the help of a railing.
Joint mobility	maintained	while on bedrest.	
The patient	will gain	1/2 oz every day.	
The patient	will lose	5 lb every week	while on a medically regulated protein diet.
Self	injection	of insulin using sterile technique by 10/12.	
The patient	will remain	afebrile during hospital stay.	

PRACTICE EXERCISE

Pick out the correctly written goal statements. Identify what is wrong with the incorrectly written goals. The answers are on the following page.

1. The patient's hydration will improve.
2. The nurse will reduce the patient's anxiety.
3. The patient will know about infant feeding.
4. Improve muscle strength.
5. 3/5: The patient will lose 6 lb in 2 weeks.
6. The patient will talk about her labor within 24 hours after delivery.
7. The decubitus ulcer (bedsore) will be healed by 2/5.
8. Verbalization of decreased pain within the next hour.
9. The patient will express confidence in her ability to breastfeed her baby before discharge.

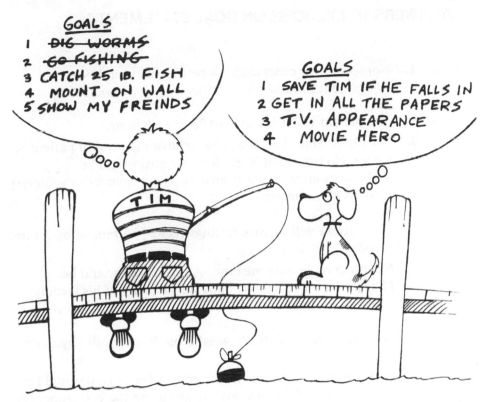

FIGURE 6. Goal setting.

10. Turn and deep breathe the patient every 2 hours.
11. Ankle edema will decrease.
12. The patient will feel better by bedtime.
13. The patient will ambulate.
14. Teach the patient AROM (active range of motion) exercises.
15. The patient's depression will improve.
16. The patient will learn about good nutrition.
17. The patient will understand the purpose of his medications before discharge.
18. The patient's temperature will stay below 101 °F during the next 24 hours.
19. The nursing student will understand the nursing process after reading this book.
20. The student will write a nursing diagnosis and a goal after finishing this chapter.

ANSWERS TO EXERCISE ON GOAL STATEMENTS

1. Not specific or observable. A better goal would be:
   The patient's intake will be 2500 cc every 24 hours.
   or
   The patient will drink at least 75 cc each hour.

2. Not observable. This is a nurse behavior instead of patient behavior. No time limit is set. A better goal would be:
   Verbalization of reduced anxiety about tomorrow's surgery by 10 p.m. tonight.
   or
   The patient will discuss feelings related to biopsy by 3 p.m. today.

3. Not observable, no time limit. A better goal would be:
   (The patient) Feeding her baby the majority of his feedings by 6/7.
   or
   Newborn regained birth weight on breast milk by 2-week checkup.

4. No subject, not specific, no criteria. A better goal would be:
   The patient will lift his own weight using the bed trapeze by 2/5.
   or
   4/5 The patient will be able to lift equal amounts of weight in 3 months with his right and his left arm.

5. O.K.

6. O.K.

7. O.K.

8. O.K. Subject (the patient) is assumed.

9. O.K.

10. This is a nursing action, not an observable patient behavior.

11. Not specific, no time limit. A better goal would be:
    Absence of pitting edema of the ankle by tomorrow at 10 p.m.
    or
    Ankle will measure less than 11 inches in circumference by tomorrow at 8 a.m.

12. Not observable. A better goal would be:
    The patient will state she feels better by 10 p.m.

13. No criteria. A better goal would be:
    The patient will walk the length of the hall by date of discharge without use of a walker.

    or

    8/2: The patient will walk from his bed to a chair in his room by tomorrow.

14. Nursing action instead of patient behavior, no time limit. A better goal would be:
    The patient will demonstrate AROM by 3 p.m. today.

    or

    The patient will have equal motion in the right and left shoulder joint by time of discharge.

15. Too vague, not observable. A better goal would be:
    The patient will sit in patient lounge for 15 minutes during this shift.

    or

    8/3: The patient will get dressed and comb her hair tomorrow a.m.

16. Not observable. A better goal would be:
    (The patient) Select a food from each of the four basic food groups for tonight's supper.

    or

    (The patient) Plan a week's menus for a low-salt diet with the help of the dietician before discharge.

17. Not observable. A better goal would be:
    The patient will state the purpose of each of his medications before discharge.

    or

    By 4/7, the patient will state route, dose, and time for each take-home medication.

18. O.K.

19. Not observable. A better goal would be:
    The nursing student will list the steps in the nursing process after reading this book.

    or

    The nursing student will write one nursing care plan after reading this book.

20. O.K.

PLANNING NURSING ACTIONS

NURSING ACTIONS:

Those things the nurse plans to do in order to help the patient achieve a goal.

Nursing actions may be thought of as instructions for all nurses caring for the patient. The attending physician will review a patient's history and care with the resident on call before leaving the hospital for the night. This is done to insure continued treatments begun by the patient's primary physician. A set of instructions to the physician on call are often part of this communication. Similarly, the nurse will leave a set of instructions for other nurses on how they might best care for a particular patient. Planned actions should be written on the care plan and numbered sequentially. This helps the nurse organize her care and ensures continuity in the patient's care from one shift to another.

Nursing orders are a form of nursing actions identifying specific care and treatments which nursing personnel have the authority to initiate for a particular patient. The care and treatments are designed to help the patient meet one or more nursing goals and thus lessen or remedy a diagnosed patient need or problem. They are often written in the form of an order on a patient's care plan, with frequency of treatment and the date clearly indicated. It is expected that other nursing personnel will follow these orders just as carefully as they would follow a physician's orders. Respect for a colleague's professional judgment is communicated by implementing her plan for patient care as outlined in a care plan. Nursing personnel are accountable for implementation and documentation of nursing orders. For example:

11/12 Urine volume q. voiding.
11/13 Ambulate q.1–2h until passing flatus.
11/12 Remove TEDS (elastic stockings) q. shift for 20 minutes.
11/11 Turn and reposition q.2h.
11/10 Catheter care b.i.d.
11/15 Warm packs to infiltrated IV site q.i.d. × 24 hours.

The following are some guidelines to review in selecting your nursing actions.

1. Nursing actions must be safe for the patient. Application of heat to the skin will stimulate circulation, but excessive heat will burn. Nursing actions using heat must ensure that the patient is not burned. Exercising a patient's muscles and joints can be very beneficial; however, if muscles and joints are forced beyond the point of resistance or pain, the nurse can cause injuries.

2. Nursing actions must be congruent with other therapies. For example, nursing actions must be selected within the safety range ordered by the physician. If the medical order reads: "Aspirin (ASA), 2 tablets, q. 4 h., p.r.n.," nursing actions cannot plan the administration of aspirin every 2 hours. If the physical therapist is instructing the patient in the use of a walker, the nurse should also use a walker in ambulating the patient.

3. Nursing actions should be based on principles and knowledge integrated from previous nursing education and experience, and from the behavioral and physical sciences. For example,

    PATIENT PROBLEM: Injury to hand with bleeding under the skin.
    PRINCIPLE: Cold constricts superficial blood vessels.
    NURSING ACTION: Apply ice pack to injured hand.

    PATIENT PROBLEM: Paralyzed and restricted to bedrest.
    PRINCIPLE: Continuous pressure on an area of skin will obstruct blood flow and may lead to tissue damage and necrosis.
    NURSING ACTIONS:
    a. Turn and reposition the patient in bed every 2 hours.
    b. Massage pressure areas every 2 hours.
    c. Alternating pressure mattress on bed.

The first courses in many nursing programs involve the student in a study of basic fundamentals of nursing practice. These fundamentals courses provide the student with the rationale for the steps of various skills and procedures in addition to teaching the motor aspects of the skill or procedure. In order to adapt nursing care to new situations, new equipment, and changing technology, the nurse must understand the rationale behind the choice of nursing actions. Principles and theories related to sterile technique, for example, have remained constant as equipment and materials changed from reusable supplies to disposable. The nurse who understands the rationale behind sterile technique for various procedures is more able to adapt nursing care to a particular patient using any variety of equipment and supplies available. Principles and theories from disciplines related to nursing, such as anatomy, physiology, psychology, and sociology, blend with nursing knowledge and experience to form an integrated base of knowledge which guides the nurse in planning patient care. While the nursing process involves an understanding of the rationale underlying nursing actions, it is not necessary to include this written rationale in documenting the care plan. However, the nursing process is incomplete and potentially unsafe unless the nurse bases her choice of nursing actions on appropriate rationale. Rationale for nursing actions is included in the various care plans in this text as a teaching tool. In clinical settings, writing rationale for nursing actions consumes much time and space and therefore is inappropriate.

The following example illustrates the principles and theories from various disciplines upon which selection of appropriate nursing actions are based.

NURSING DIAGNOSIS: Pain related to cervical dilation of labor.

NURSING GOAL: Patient verbalizations related to coping successfully with the discomfort of labor.

Nursing Actions	*Rationale*
a. Encourage husband to stay with wife, if desired by the couple.	a. When individuals are under stress, presence of their support system can reduce the effects of stress.
b. Assess frequently for signs of muscle tension. Encourage relaxation through massage, heat, cold, and slow breathing when possible.	b. Fear can lead to increased muscle tension. Increased muscle tension can lead to increased perception of pain. Continuous muscle tension depletes energy reserves. Massage of tense muscles may help individuals to relax those muscles. Heat or cold may feel soothing as labor progresses

c. Keep couple informed of progress. Encourage questions; explanations.

d. Assist with breathing techniques learned for labor.

e. Encourage use of a focal point.

f. Offer technique of effleurage.

g. Verbal encouragement and praise for efforts to manage discomfort of labor.

h Request order for analgesics p.r.n.

i. Assess cervical dilation and fetal heart rate before administering any analgesics.

and aid relaxation. Muscle tension can be reduced as patients consciously relax while slowly exhaling.

c. Fear may be caused by insufficient or inaccurate information.

d. Individuals can be conditioned to respond to a stimulus with specific learned behavior. Distraction can help lessen pain perception. Practice with feedback leads to improved performance.

e. Visual concentration may distract from pain perception.

f. Tactile stimulation can interfere with deeper pain sensations.

g. Positive reinforcement of desired behavior increases the occurrence of that behavior.

h. Chemical agents alter the perception of pain.

i. Analgesics given late in labor may depress the fetus at birth. Cervical dilation may change rapidly in the active phase of labor. Fetal heart rate is an indicator of fetal well-being. Analgesics given to the mother can further depress a compromised fetus.

4. Write one set of nursing actions to accomplish each goal.

5. Choose a set of nursing actions most likely to develop the behavior described in the goal statement. There may be many different nursing actions which would accomplish the same goal. The nurse should attempt to give the patient practice in the specific behavior stated in the goal.

   NURSING DIAGNOSIS: Pain related to bone cancer.

   NURSING GOAL: Verbalization related to experiencing minimal pain during hospitalization.

Nursing Actions/Orders	
May Achieve Goal	*More Likely to Achieve Goal*
a. Offer prescribed pain medication q. 3–4 h.	a. Assess patient's pain, timing, duration, intensity, and related activities.
b. Assist patient with ADL	b. Assess patient's current methods of dealing with pain and support as possible.
	c. Discuss and practice alternate pain relief measures with patient. (1) relaxation (2) alternative sensory stimulation —music —tactile (massage, effleurage, menthol rubs, vibrators) —heat/cold —movies, TV, reading (3) breathing techniques
	d. Discuss self-medication for pain.
	e. Discuss effectiveness of pain relief measures with physician and patient.
	f. Encourage use of pain relief measures when discomfort *begins* rather than after it is intense.

6. Nursing actions should be realistic:
   —for the patient. Consider age, physical strength, disease, willingness to change behavior, resources.
   —for the number of hospital staff. Will enough people consistently be available to carry out the nursing actions?
   —for the experience and ability of available staff. If most of the staff are unfamiliar with the nursing actions you are suggesting, there is a high probability they will not be carried out.
   —for available equipment. If your nursing actions include the use of any equipment, it should be readily available and the hospital staff should be familiar with its use.

7. Whenever possible, nursing actions should be important to the patient and compatible with personal goals and values. The patient should understand how the nursing actions will result in achievement of the goal. For example, a child may not understand the importance of good nutrition to his recovery, but he might love to play games. If the nursing actions can make a game out of eating, the child may begin to eat more because he values the eating game the nurse has created. An adult may refuse to do arm and hand exercises because he does not think they are important. If the nursing actions encourage the patient to do activities such as shaving, combing his hair, brushing his teeth, and feeding himself, the arms and hands will still receive the desired exercise. The difference is that the patient values being able to do these self-care activities and can see that they are part of his recovery.

8. Use the patient as a source for choosing nursing actions. The patient may have many good suggestions for activities he can use to achieve a certain goal based on his past experience. The nurse can use her knowledge and experience to incorporate some of the patient's suggestions into the nursing actions she will write for this patient's care plan. This will help to involve the patient in planning his own care. The more involved the patient is and the more he values the goal, the more he will cooperate with his care.

> NURSING DIAGNOSIS: Dehydration related to diarrhea.
> MEDICAL ORDER: Diet: Force clear fluids
> GOAL: Patient will have an oral intake of 1500 cc for 10/22.

> NURSING ACTIONS: NURSING ACTIONS:
>
> *Nurse A*   *Nurse B*
> a. Offer water q. 2 h.   a. Explain goal to patient.
> b. Record intake.   b. Ask patient what he likes to drink.
>   c. Offer favorite clear fluid q. 2 h.
>   d. Show patient how to record intake and keep track of progress toward goal.

9. List nursing actions sequentially. Generally there will be several planned actions for each goal statement. Many times, one action is dependent on a previous action. By listing these

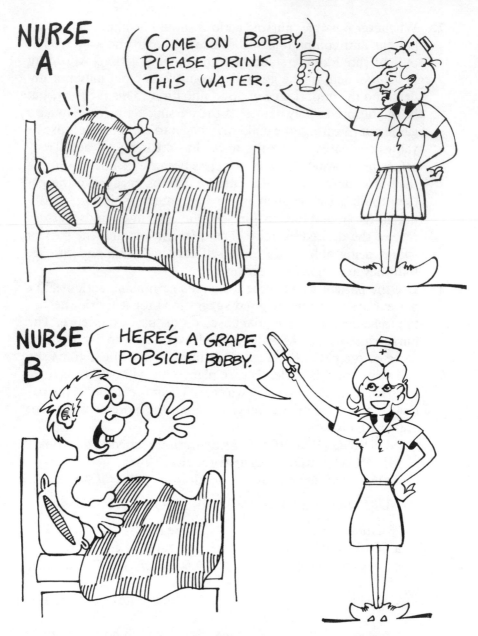

FIGURE 7.   Whenever possible, nursing actions should take the patient's preferences into account.

actions in the order in which they should occur, the nursing staff knows the sequence that should be used in giving care to this patient. The implications of the following factors should be considered when ordering nursing actions.

> *Maslow's hierarchy*—meeting lower level survival needs before higher level needs may enable your patient to function at his optimal level. For example, the following sequence of nursing actions deals with the lower need of pain avoidance before asking the patient to deal with actions to prevent complications.

NURSING DIAGNOSIS: Prone to respiratory complications following surgery with general anesthesia.

NURSING GOAL: Normal respiratory functioning within 24 hours post-op.

NURSING ACTIONS:

    a. Explain goal to patient.

    b. Explain preventive function of the following activities.

        (1) Turning, coughing, and deep breathing at least every 2 hours.

        (2) Early ambulation.

        (3) Use of deep breathing device.

    c. Explain ways to minimize discomfort during turning and coughing.

    d. Offer pain medication 1/2 hour prior to ambulating.

    e. Assist patient to: (Nursing Orders)

        (1) TCH q. 2 h.

        (2) Ambulate q.i.d. starting first post-op day.

        (3) Deep breather q. 1 h while awake.

> *Medical Orders*—some medical orders may require nursing activities, such as patient assessment, prior to carrying out the physician's order, to insure patient safety. For example:

MEDICAL ORDER: Lanoxin 0.125 mg q.d.

NURSING ACTION:

    a. Count apical pulse *prior* to *every* medication administration.

    b. Give Lanoxin 0.125 mg. at 8 a.m. q.d. if pulse above 60 beats per minute. Hold if pulse significantly above previously recorded rate or below 60 beats per minute.

   c. Notify physician if medication held.

MEDICAL ORDER: Magnesium sulfate 5 gm deep IM q. 6 h.

NURSING ACTIONS:

   a. Assess patient's reflexes, urine output, and respiratory rate *prior* to *every* medication administration.

   b. Give $MgSO_4$ 5 gm deep IM at $8^A-2^P-8^P-2^A$ if reflexes normal or brisk. Hold medication and consult physician if reflexes depressed or absent; if urine output less than 30 cc per hour, or if respirations are below 12 breaths per minute.

Scientific principles—These will often guide the sequence of the activities in various nursing skills.

Patient preferences

Hospital routine

Developing a Teaching Plan

If the nurse assesses a patient and makes a nursing diagnosis related to a knowledge or performance deficit, a teaching plan will most likely comprise a large portion of the activity in the planning phase of the nursing process. Inadequate or incorrect knowledge may also be related to various other patient problems. Unrealistic fears of a medical procedure or incorrectly administered prescribed medications are examples that could be caused by the patient's belief in erroneous information. Patients with newly diagnosed medical problems are frequently confronted with knowledge deficits concerning the implications of their medical diagnosis and the effect it may have on their life style. Patients taking on new roles, such as parenting, are frequently concerned about their lack of knowledge and skill in newborn care. Prenatal classes such as Lamaze and CEA will anticipate these learning needs and identify specific areas of newborn care that various groups would like to discuss in class. Nursing follow-through in the hospital, after delivery, builds on this information and gives the parents actual practice in caring for their newborn. Similarly, preoperative and postoperative teaching is based on a nursing diagnosis related to inadequate knowledge of postsurgical complications and preventive measures. Preoperative teaching is also based on research indicating that an educated patient, knowing what will happen during a procedure, will often experience less pain and anxiety than an unprepared patient. The nursing diagnosis, again, would relate to inadequate or incorrect information about a particular procedure or surgery.

In applying the nursing process to the formulation of a teaching plan, the nurse follows a logical sequence of problem solving. First, she identifies the knowledge deficit in the assessment phase of the nursing process. A goal is then chosen which identifies the learning outcomes. Next, a plan is developed to teach the skill or information to the patient. There are two basic types of learning outcomes which will be discussed in this text: the accomplishment of a specific goal and the accomplishment of more generalized goals incorporating specific ones.

In the first type, the nurse may find a rather specific area in which the patient needs information in order to understand or perform a particular activity. An example of this would be a newly delivered primipara who does not know how to take a rectal temperature on her newborn.

NURSING DIAGNOSIS: Lack of knowledge in taking newborn rectal temperature.

GOAL: Take an accurate rectal temperature on her newborn before discharge.

PLAN:
1. Demonstrate how to take rectal temperatures on newborns.
2. Explain safety precautions and when to notify physician for fevers.
3. Provide reinforced practice in taking her newborn's temperature.

Another example would be a patient with a nursing diagnosis of "confusion related to self-administration of medication."

GOAL: Demonstrate correct self-administration of medication by 11/3.

PLAN:
1. Discuss with the patient how to safely take each medication (drug, dose, time, route).
2. Supervise patient in hospital with self-administration of prescribed medications.
3. Provide a clear set of directions in written form regarding medications.
4. Check that patient can read all labels on medications.

When patients need to learn specific motor skills, the stated goal has a very direct relationship to the diagnosed knowledge or performance deficit. The teaching plan and eventually the evaluation of the patient's ability to perform the skill are usually equally specific. The nurse follows the steps of the nursing process when she:

1. Identifies knowledge deficit (NURSING DIAGNOSIS).

2. Identifies the specific behavior the patient will perform based
    on the diagnosed learning need (GOAL).
3. Teaches the specific behavior to the patient (PLAN).
4. Tests the patient's ability to perform the specific behavior
    (EVALUATION).

Evaluating patient learning may be difficult if observable behaviors are not identified as learning objectives during the planning phase. This direct approach may be inappropriate for teaching patients with more generalized learning needs. When a patient is developing an understanding of broader concepts or improving cognitive skills, the nurse's teaching plan cannot focus on one specific behavior as evidence of this broader understanding. For example, if the diagnosis relates to inadequate knowledge of infant care, a goal dealing with the isolated behavior of diapering does not provide support for the assumption that the parent is competent in infant care. In this case, the method the nurse may use is the identification of one broader learning goal and then subsequent identification of several specific goals which are examples of

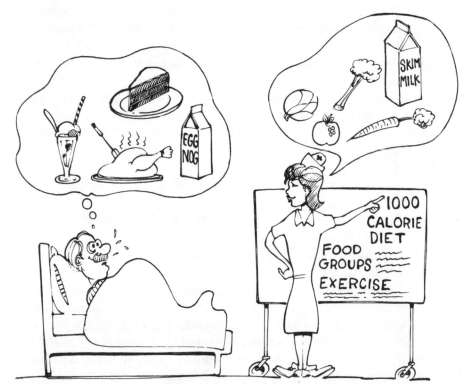

FIGURE 8. A good teaching plan does not always guarantee that patient
learning will occur.

the broader goal. The broader goal may be difficult to state in behavioral terms. The examples of specific goals should be stated as observable or measurable behaviors. The teaching plan is then directed at the broader goal while including the specific goals.

Example 1:

NURSING DIAGNOSIS: Inadequate knowledge and skill related to newborn care.

NURSING GOAL: Parents will safely care for newborn by time of discharge from hospital.

BROAD GOAL: May not be observable.

SPECIFIC GOALS: Should be observable.

1. Demonstrate bathing their newborn.
2. Safely take a rectal temperature on newborn.
3. Demonstrate cord care for umbilical stump.
4. Breast-feeding: 10–15 minutes per breast q. 2–5 h.
5. Bring infant car seat for transporting newborn home from hospital.

TEACHING PLAN: Nursing actions

1. Assess readiness for learning infant care. (Comfort level, fatigue, personal priority needs)
2. Discuss various aspects of infant care: feedings, hygiene, safety, growth and development, behavior.
3. Demonstrate specific infant care skills and provide practice for parents with positive reinforcement.
4. Assist in initiation of breast-feeding and provide specific information on the skill.
5. Provide resources for parents after discharge. (People to call when questions or problems arise)

Example 2:

NURSING DIAGNOSIS: Inadequate knowledge related to the nursing process.

NURSING GOAL: Student will understand and utilize the nursing process in providing patient care.

BROAD GOAL: May not be observable

SPECIFIC GOALS: Observable

1. Identify four phases of the nursing process.
2. Explain nursing diagnosis and how it differs from medical diagnosis.
3. Write three nursing diagnoses from a data base.
4. Write three nursing goals with subject, verb, and criteria of performance.

    5. Write three sets of nursing actions to help a patient meet specific goals.

    6. Evaluate goal achievement and reassess care plan.

TEACHING PLAN: Nursing Actions

1. Discuss rationale for using the nursing process.
2. Explain, briefly, the relationship between the nursing process and patient care.
3. Assign readings on nursing process.
4. Demonstrate application of nursing process on a hypothetical patient's data base.
5. Use practice exercises for writing nursing diagnoses, goals, and planning actions.
6. Written student assignment: Develop a care plan on your assigned hospital patient showing assessment, planning, implementation, and evaluation.
7. Review and critique students' care plans.

There are several things to consider when developing a teaching plan. Learning is enhanced by using principles of teaching learning. It is especially important to assess the patient's readiness to learn. An illness, medical problem, or treatment may greatly interfere with learning, particularly in the acute phase of an illness. Medications, fatigue, motivation, anxiety, pain, or hunger may all block effective learning. Teaching should be delayed until some of these obstacles have been lessened or eliminated. The nurse also needs to assess the patient's previous knowledge and skills, building on this prior base. Begin at the level of patient understanding using language clear to the patient. Individualizing the teaching approach may also lead to improved patient learning. The following principles applied to health teaching may be helpful.

Common Components of a Teaching Plan	Rationale and Scientific Principles
1. Setting a learning goal with the patient.	1. Clarification of desired learning outcomes will guide teaching methods and may serve as a motivating function for the learner.

2. Assessing patient's readiness to learn.
  a. motivation
  b. illness/medical problem
  c. medication/pain
  d. level of consciousness
	2. A person learns more effectively when the learning experience has personal relevance. A person learns more effectively when a need to learn is perceived.

e. anxiety level
f. fatigue

Unmet physical or psychosocial needs such as anxiety,
pain, and fatigue have a nega-
tive effect on attention, reten-
tion, and ability to learn.

3. Assess patient's current knowledge and motor skill ability.
4. Begin teaching at the patient's
current level of understanding or
skill performance.

3., 4. Teaching which moves from
simple to complex will help to
ensure understanding. Simple
and complex are relative
terms and have meaning only
in relationship to the learner's
current level of understanding
or performance.

5. Provide the patient with an opportunity to practice motor skills
after a demonstration.
6. Reinforce patient's efforts to
learn whenever possible.

5., 6. An active learner learns and
retains more than a passive
learner. Practice with feedback and positive reinforcement leads to improved performance and continuance of
reinforced behavior.

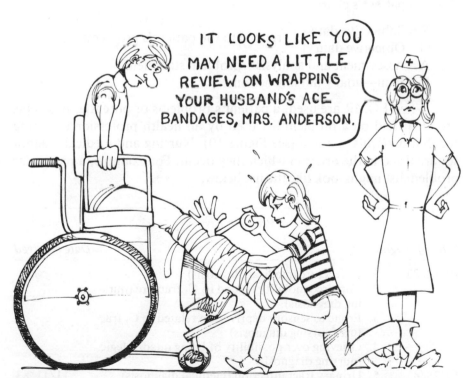

FIGURE 9.   Assess your patient's or family member's ability to perform a
skill and build on prior learning.

DOCUMENTATION OF PATIENT CARE

By the end of the planning phase of the nursing process, the nurse is ready to begin direct patient care. Nurses must document the quality of patient care which results from consistent use of the nursing process. The patient's nursing care plan should be a part of the permanent record as are the plans of other health professionals caring for individuals requiring their special expertise. Listed here are several ways in which this may be accomplished.

1. Writing quality care plans which then become part of the permanent patient record upon patient discharge. This option may necessitate some changes in current care plan forms to allow more room for the nurse's diagnoses, goals, plan, and evaluation. This is currently a practice in some hospitals.

2. Use of Problem Oriented Medical Records (POMR) with charting done in a format which allows documentation of most of the steps in the nursing process. This is referred to as SOAP charting. All members of the health care team follow this format when documenting information in a patient's chart.

$$S = \text{Subjective data} \left.\right\} \text{ related to the patient's problems}$$
$$O = \text{Objective data}$$
A = Assessment and analysis—problem statement
P = Plan—goal + nursing actions

When POMR are used, a patient's problems or potential problems are identified on a problem list used by all health professionals caring for that particular patient (see Figure 10). Nursing and medical diagnoses are listed in the order in which they occur. For example, a particular problem list might look like the list below.

Problem List

Date of diagnosis		Date resolved
10/12/83	1. C_5 fracture (medical diagnosis)	
	2. Impaired mobility related to C_5 fracture (nursing diagnosis)	
	3. Prone to sensory deprivation related to C_5 fracture (nursing diagnosis)	
	4. Grieving over possibility of being quadriplegic (nursing diagnosis)	
10/28/83	5. Urinary tract infection (medical diagnosis)	11/11/83

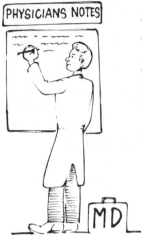

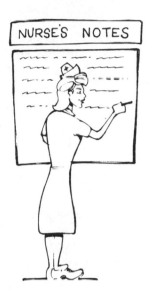

Traditional documenta-
tion in patient's charts
may block communica-
tion and understanding
among health care
professionals.

POMR may help improve
communication among
health care professionals.

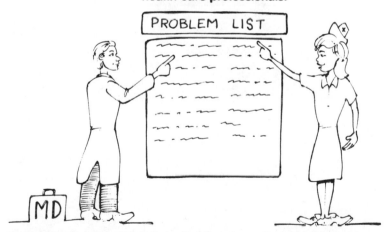

FIGURE 10. Traditional documentation versus the POMR.

SOAP charting would then deal with a specific problem in a consistent method to assure complete documentation. For example, in problem 2:

S: "I can only shrug my shoulders. I can't move my arms or legs. I can't feel anything below my shoulders."
O: On circle bed with crutchfield tongs and 10 lb weight. No voluntary movement in extremities and trunk.
A: Prone to complications of immobility.
P: The patient will experience no preventable complications of immobility.

1. Turn and reposition q. 2 h.
2. Passive ROM exercises to all extremities q.i.d.
3. Massage pressure points q. 2 h.
4. Circle bed for maintenance of body alignment.
5. TEDS (elastic stockings to groin).
6. Oral intake above 1500 cc per day. Offer fluids q. 2 h.
7. Encourage visitors, use of phone, roommate to prevent social isolation.

3. Use of SOAPIE(R) charting for nursing: This is an alternative to SOAP charting. It includes three more steps and follows more completely the application of the nursing process to patient care. This detail might be most appropriate as a summary note on the chart for evaluation of the nursing goals identified in the care plan. This type of entry may not be appropriate until after the implementation phase of the nursing process.

    S = Subjective data
    O = Objective data
    A = Assessment
    P = Plan
    I = Implementation or Intervention to carry out the plan
    E = Evaluation of plan
    (R) = Reassessment of patient's need and nursing plan (This step may be included in evaluation in the guidelines for charting in some institutions.)

CASE STUDY: MRS. SMITH PLANNING PHASE

NURSING CARE PLAN WORKSHEET

PATIENT: Mrs. Smith

Nursing Diagnosis	Goals	Planned Action	Rationale
1. Inadequate information related to diabetes mellitus.	1. Understanding of self-care needs associated with diabetes as evidenced by performing the following before discharge: —Planning a 3 day menu for her family which meets diabetic diet requirements. —Listing signs and symptoms of hyperglycemia/hypoglycemia. —Correctly performing diabetic urine testing. —Performing daily diabetic foot care. —Correctly explaining how to cope with short-term illness while managing her diabetes.	1. a. Assess learning readiness. b. Begin teaching when patient shows signs of acceptance of medical diagnosis. Include family, as possible. c. Referral to dietitian for diabetic diet teaching and evaluation. d. Assess understanding of diabetes. Build on patient's current knowledge. e. Discuss diabetes: etiology, treatment, and prognosis.	1. a. Anxiety, fear, and discomfort can interfere with learning. b. Denial of initial diagnosis may occur in grief response over lost "health." c. Most appropriate professional. d. Beginning teaching at the learner's level improves understanding. Learning which moves from simple to complex increases understanding. e. Providing accurate knowledge base aids individuals in problem solving and may allay unrealistic fears.

—Demonstrating competence in self-administration of oral hypoglycemia med.
—Explaining actions to take for hyperglycemia/hypoglycemia.
—Purchasing medic alert tag.

f. Explain rationale and demonstrate diabetic foot care q.d. at h.s. × 2. Encourage self-care thereafter.

g. Explain and demonstrate diabetic urine testing q.i.d. Encourage self-testing when patient feels ready.

h. Explain dietary and activity interrelationships and relationship to hyperglycemia/hypoglycemia.

i. Discuss signs, symptoms, and treatment for hyperglycemia/hypoglycemia.

j. Discuss short-term illness; effect on diabetic management.

f., g. Learning is facilitated when a need to learn is perceived. Learning is enhanced by active participation. Demonstration and explanation utilize 2 modes of communication and improve comprehension.

h. Increased activity and decreased food intake may predispose diabetic to hypoglycemia. Decreased activity and increased food consumption may predispose diabetic to hyperglycemia.

i. Early treatment of hyper/hypoglycemia can prevent more severe complications.

j. Illness, fever, nausea, diarrhea can lead to hypoglycemia.

Nursing Diagnosis	Goals	Planned Action	Rationale
		k. Provide reference list on diabetes.	k. Identifying references for further learning offers learners options in meeting personal needs when ready.
		l. Explain rationale for medic alert tag and how to order.	l. Knowledge of diabetic condition will affect medical care if an emergency should occur, and patient unable to communicate.
2. Fear related to possible complications of diabetes.	2. Fear of complications to be based on verbalizations of accurate data regarding progress and complications of adult onset diabetes mellitus by discharge.	2. a. Assess understanding of complications and preventive measures. Include family whenever possible.	2. a. Learning is facilitated when a need to learn is perceived. Learning which moves from simple to complex increases learner comprehension. Positive reinforcement by significant others will increase the appearance of reinforced behavior.

b. Build on prior knowledge in the following areas, including signs and symptoms, prevention and treatment.
   (1) Skin complications
   (2) Periodontal disease
   (3) Visual problems

b. (1) Increased glucose pooling in epidermis predisposes diabetics to infection. Glucose is a growth medium for bacteria.
   (2) Diabetics are more prone to periodontal disease resulting in bone loss around teeth.
   (3) Changing glucose levels can affect the lens of the eye and decrease visual activity. Elevated glucose levels predispose the diabetic to cataract formation. Glaucoma may be more prevalent in diabetics. Diabetics are prone to micro-aneurysms in the retina. Rupture can obstruct vision.

Nursing Diagnosis	Goals	Planned Action	Rationale
		(4) Heart disease	(4) Diabetes is a risk factor for arteriosclerotic heart disease.
		(5) Vascular problem	(5) Diabetics are prone to arterial insufficiency, especially in extremities.
		(6) Kidney, bladder problems	(6) Diabetes may cause changes in glomerular filtration. Waste products may accumulate in the blood.
		(7) Neuropathies	(7) Atrophy of small muscles in hands, sensory impairment in extremities, diarrhea and constipation, bladder and reproductive dysfunction may all be signs and symptoms of diabetic neuropathies.

c. Provide printed material for follow-up teaching.

d. Discuss patient concerns and teaching done with other members of health teams.

e. Suggest possible support groups with other diabetics to discuss concerns.

c. Multiple communication modes will increase the clarity of the message (teaching).

d. Communication from various health professionals, which builds on previous teaching improves patient's understanding. Follow-up visits can reinforce learned patient behavior and increase occurrence of goal behaviors.

e. Anxiety and unmet needs can interfere with learning and willingness to follow suggested medical treatment. Verbalization of concerns with others who are perceived as able to understand can lead to successful resolution of fear, anger, and frustration.

Nursing Diagnosis	Goals	Planned Action	Rationale
3. Altered body image related to diagnosis of diabetes mellitus.	3. Verbalizations of feelings related to diabetes indicating positive self-concept by 11/12.	3. a. Assess her understanding of diabetic condition as explained by physician.	3. a. Building on communication from other professionals in the health team reinforces and clarifies the message. Anxiety can distort understanding of a message.
		b. Share possible reactions of grief response and effect on self-concept.	b. Loss of previously perceived "healthy state" often results in grief responses. Feelings of isolation or abnormality in reaction to loss may interfere with successful adaptation to new physical state. Guilt and self-blame may accompany grief reactions.
		c. Encourage expression of feelings related to her diagnosis.	c. Verbalizations of concerns and feelings can lead to successful resolution of fear, anger, frustration.

4. Prone to hyperglycemia related to family and personal eating patterns.

Short-Term: Plan a 3-day menu for self and her family which meets diabetic diet requirements.
Long-Term: Prevention of severe hyperglycemia after discharge from hospital. (4+ or 2% urine glucose)

d. Discuss possible reactions she anticipates or observes in her family related to her diagnosis. Include family if possible.

e. Discuss realistic limitations imposed by her condition.

4. a. Referral to dietician for diet teaching.

b. Encourage public health nurse referral first week at home.

c. Provide both referrals with data regarding patient and family eating patterns.

d. Fears of rejection or inadequacy in relationships with significant others can threaten love/belonging and self-esteem needs. Validation of family's actual reactions will provide accurate data for problem-solving.

e. Abilities focus facilitates restoration of self-esteem.

4. a. Most appropriate professional.

b. Follow-up visit by member of health team can reinforce learned patient behaviors. Application of learning may lead to questions, uncertainty, etc., which an early home visit can alleviate.

c. Building on patient's prior eating patterns and habits will personalize teaching and assist in identifying

Nursing Diagnosis	Goals	Planned Action	Rationale
		d. Plan family conference to discuss dangers of hyperglycemia and causative eating patterns. Help family negotiate new eating patterns to lessen risks of hyperglycemia.	potential problems. Starting at patient's level and moving to more unfamiliar material will facilitate learning.
			d. Active involvement facilitates learning and mutual support. Individualizing eating patterns to meet preferences of various family members may facilitate cooperation with new menus.
		e. Review signs and symptoms of hyperglycemia with patient and family. Discuss steps to take in diagnosing the problem before blood levels of glucose cause problems requiring hospitalization.	e. Knowledge of problems and their prevention by all family members may allay unrealistic fears and give members a feeling of control.

5. Prone to skin infection related to diabetes and overweight.

5. Absence of skin infections during hospitalization and after discharge.

f. Discuss need for medical care if hyperglycemia becomes severe–who to call, where to go, a.m. or p.m.

g. Follow-up phone call 2 days after discharge and 2 weeks after discharge to discuss adjustments.

5. a. Assess patient's understanding of diabetic skin care and rationale for increased incidence of infection.

b. Build on prior knowledge of skin care and personal grooming preferences.

c. Review with patient:
(1) Skin areas most likely to become infected or irritated.

f. Anticipatory problem-solving may reduce stress and inappropriate behavior in an actual emergency.

g. Same as 4.b. above.

5. a. Learning is facilitated when a need to learn is perceived. Learning which moves from simple to complex increases learner comprehension.

b. The learner's interest and motivation increases when the learning experience has personal relevance.

c. (1) Diabetics have excess glucose pooling under epidermis, particularly in areas of axilla, breasts, and groin.

Nursing Diagnosis	Goals	Planned Action	Rationale
		(2) Signs and symptoms which may indicate infection starting.	(2) Skin may become "beefy red" or purple-red, especially from Candida albicans; Pustular lesions and oozing.
		(3) Prevention of bacterial growth.	(3) Brownish areas may indicate extensive blood vessel changes in diabetic. Shin spots may result from trauma. High moisture, body heat, darkness, and excess cutaneous glucose facilitates bacterial growth. Frequent bathing and keeping adjacent skin surfaces dry will inhibit this tendency in diabetics. Cotton underwear allows evaporation of moisture.

(4) Importance of balanced diet and maintaining ideal weight.

    (4) Well-nourished tissue is more resistant to trauma and heals more rapidly. Excess weight causes irritation from rubbing of skin surfaces.

d. Nursing orders:

(1) Foot care q.d. 9 p.m.

d. (1) Diabetics are prone to decreased blood circulation in their feet and healing problems. Loss of sensation, muscle atrophy, and bone changes can occur in the diabetic foot.

(2) Shower or tub q.d.

    (2) Frequent bathing decreases bacteria and accumulated glucose.

(3) Cornstarch or powder under breasts b.i.d.

    (3) Powder absorbs moisture and reduces friction of adjacent skin surfaces.

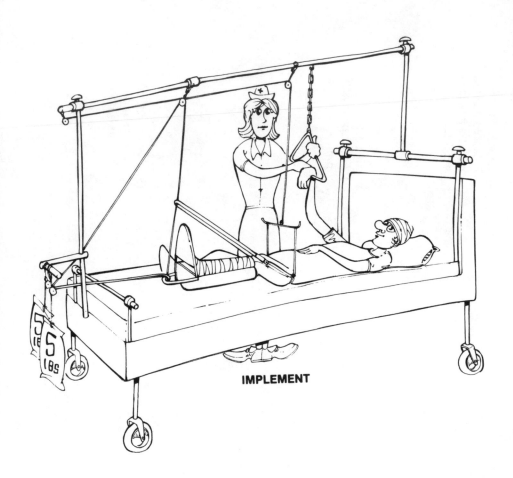

IMPLEMENT

CHAPTER 3

Implementation

Like the other steps comprising the nursing process, the implementation phase consists of several activities: validating the care plan, writing the care plan, giving nursing care, and continuing to collect data.

Implementation = Validating Care Plan + Documenting Care Plan + Giving Nursing Care + Continuing Data Collection

VALIDATING THE CARE PLAN

When the nursing student or inexperienced staff nurse writes a care plan, it is recommended that she take the proposed care plan to a colleague and request validation. This step does not have to involve a lengthy scheduled consultation but is, rather, a very brief time during which she seeks the opinion of another nurse. It is important that the student seek appropriate sources for validation. For example, the student may request her clinical instructor or team leader to review her care plan. Such qualified sources can evaluate the care plan by using the following questions as guides.

1. Does the plan assure the patient's safety?
2. Is the plan based on sound scientific principles?

3.   Is the plan supported by accepted nursing knowledge?
4.   Are the nursing diagnoses supported by the data?
5.   Does the goal relate to the problem identified in the nursing diagnosis?
6.   Does the goal contain a time and patient behavior for evaluation?
7.   Can the planned nursing actions realistically assist the patient to achieve the intended goal?
8.   Are the nursing actions arranged in a logical sequence?
9.   Is the plan individualized to the needs and capabilities of this particular patient?
10. Are the patient's priorities being considered?

Thus, the nurse who provides the validation is reviewing the plan in two major areas:

1.   Sound nursing practice
2.   Individualized nursing care

Because of their expertise in nursing care, other nurses are the most frequently used validating professionals. At times, a nurse may wish to utilize another health team member to review some aspect of a nursing care plan. For example, the nurse teaching a diabetic client about a diabetic exchange diet may wish to have a dietician validate food substitutions requested by the patient.

Occasionally, a nursing student may select an inappropriate person to validate a care plan. Frequently, nurse aides are very knowledgeable about a specific type of care, having had several years' experience in a particular clinical area. However, the nursing student should not ask the aide to validate a care plan. The nurse aide may be a source for data in that she may be able to provide information about routines of the clinical area, but the nurse aide is not a planner of nursing care. This is a function of the nurse.

Having reviewed the plan with another professional, the student or nurse may wish to share the completed plan with the patient, who is another possible source for validation. The patient can advise the nurse if any aspect of the plan is unacceptable. Not all goals and plans are shared by the nurse and patient but agreement is desirable whenever possible. This gives the patient another opportunity to participate in planning his own care. In summary, to validate the plan is to request another appropriate professional and the patient, if possible, to give the plan approval for implementation.

DOCUMENTING THE NURSING CARE PLAN

To retain a nursing care plan for the exclusive use of one nurse is to defeat a primary purpose of care plans. In order to get the maximum effect, a care plan must get the maximum press!

A nurse may plan a patient care conference as a "press conference" for a completed care plan. At such a meeting the nurse summarizes data, problems, goals, and planned actions. She spends most of the time focusing on presenting the care plan to the team. At such a time the nurse may also gain new information from team members to add to the care plan. This conference may also be used as a problem solving session during which a nurse may request assistance from colleagues to further develop a care plan.

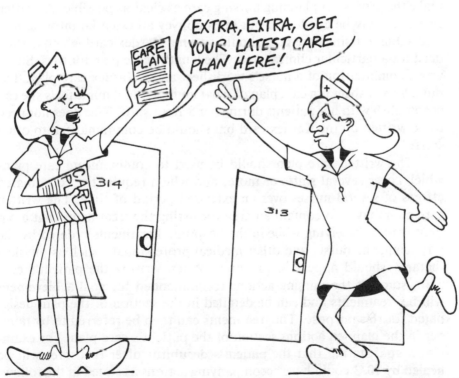

FIGURE 11. A nursing care plan must be shared, in order to be effective.

Another communication tool is the written care plan. In many hospitals, both physicians and nurses utilize a type of documentation known as problem oriented medical records (POMR). The care plan in such a system then takes the form of SOAP or SOAPIER notes as discussed in Chapter 2 of this text. Many hospitals also utilize a nursing Kardex as a system of organizing care plans. A nursing Kardex is a file which contains the care plans for a group of patients. Each plan is usually written on 6 × 11 inch index cards. Most hospitals have special forms designed for this purpose. The form may vary, but it should be a useful tool for communicating care plans. Most Kardexes will include space for nursing diagnoses, goals, nursing actions, and evaluations. Some health care settings are beginning to require that the care plan be written in ink and retained as a part of patients' permanent legal records to further document nursing care. Some hospitals have adopted 8½ × 11 inch nursing care plan forms which have the advantage of corresponding to standard chart size. Most Kardex cards give space for only an abbreviated form of the nursing care plan. In Chapter 2 (PLANNING), Mrs. Smith's care plan was written out completely to make the process of planning nursing care as clear as possible. A written care plan may be condensed but must convey all essential information. The actual nursing care plan should fit on a Kardex card which is standard for a particular clinical area. The lengthy care plan for Mrs. Smith was a combination of a nurse's worksheet and a Kardex care plan. The nurse's worksheet is a care plan of what an individual nurse feels she can accomplish with her patients during her 8-hour shift. This does not need to be written on the Kardex card but should be communicated to other staff.

The written care plan should be used to communicate care plans which cover several shifts or more, and which require the coordinated efforts of several nurses over an extended period of time. The written care plan may also contain an area for listing the treatments that a patient is to be receiving while in the hospital. Treatments ordered by the physician, the nurse, and other medical professionals, such as physical therapy, should appear in this area. When writing the patient's care plan, some of the nursing actions recommended for goal achievement will be treatments and can be detailed in the section of the plan designated for this purpose. The treatments can then be referred to by number in the planned actions section of the patient's care plan. For example, a goal stating that the patient's decubitus ulcer (bedsore) will be healed by 10/3 could have accompanying actions as stated in the following form.

Treatment or Nursing Orders	*Planned Actions*
1. Clean decubitus ulcer b.i.d. c̄ hydrogen peroxide.	1. Explain treatments and rationale to patient.
2. Turn and reposition q. 2 h.	2. Keep patient off ulcer area.
3. Apply heat lamp to ulcer b.i.d. for 10 min.	3. Encourage adequate diet and fluids.
4. Whirlpool bath to ulcer q.d.	4. Tx. 1–5.
5. Massage area around ulcer q. 2 h.	

The following suggestions will assist the nurse to write a care plan on a Kardex or any similar form.

1. Category headings should include nursing diagnoses, goals, nursing actions, and evaluations.
2. Abbreviate whenever possible, using standardized medical or English symbols.
3. Choose key words to communicate ideas; do not write whole sentences.
4. Refer people to procedure books rather than trying to include all the steps for a procedure on a written plan.
5. Include a date for evaluation of each goal.
6. When goals are met or changed, indicate the evaluation of each goal. Hospital policy may require that goals which are discontinued are signed by the responsible nurse.
7. The nursing diagnosis with the related goal and nursing actions should appear next to each other on the care plan.
8. All long-term goals should be written. Nursing actions directly related to long-term goals should also be written. If a short-term goal will be evaluated within the nurse's 8-hour shift, it is not necessary to include it on the written form. It is necessary to document the nursing care.
9. Short-term goals which cannot be met within an 8-hour shift should be written in order that other nurses can continue the plan of care.
10. Long-term goals being met by a series of short-term goals do not have accompanying written nursing actions. Write the current progressive short-term goal and its accompanying actions in any manner which clearly indicates the relationship to the long-term goal. If the short-term goal is to be met by the nurse writing the care plan, she should write the next progressive short-term goal and nursing actions (see Figure 12).

ABBREVIATED CARE PLAN

Admitted: 11/6
Discharged: 11/16

PATIENT: Mrs. Smith

Nursing Diagnosis	Goals	Date taught	Planned Action	Evaluation
11/9 Inadeq. info./ diabetes.	Understanding of self-care needs associated c̄ diabetes by discharge. Pt. to demonstrate:		1. Assess knowledge and learning readiness.	
Prone to hyperglycemia related to family and personal eating patterns.	a. Short-term: 3-day menu planning. Long-term: Prevention of 4+/2% urine glucose after discharge.	11/12 D. Smith R.D.	2. Teaching plan to incorporate all of specific goals. 3. Dietetic referral 11/10.	
	b. Info of signs/symptoms and remedy for hyper/ hypoglycemia.	11/11 K. Ray R.N.	4. Provide references on diabetes when she is ready.	
	c. Diabetic urine testing.	11/10 J. Line R.N.	5. Public health referral for follow-up evaluation.	
	d. Diabetic foot care.	11/11 K. Ray R.N.		
Prone to skin infec./diabetes and overweight.	e. Diabetic skin care; absence of skin infec.	11/10 J. Line R.N.		
	f. Self-administration of meds.	11/11 K. Ray R.N.		
	g. Info. for coping c̄ short-term illness.	11/13 D. Adams R.N.		
	h. Purchase of medic alert tag.	11/13 D. Adams R.N.		

78

Fears possible complications of diabetes.	Fears of complications based on accurate data by 11/12.	1. Individualized teaching plan. 2. Family conference—feelings/concerns. 3. Offer community support groups.
Altered body image/diabetes.	Verbalizations of positive self-image by 11/12.	1. Assess reaction to dx. 2. Discuss possible grief response. 3. Discuss family reactions. 4. Realistic limitations—abilities focus.

Medications

Diabinase 250 mg q.d. 7 a.m.

Nursing Orders/Tx.

diabetic urines q.i.d. 6-11-4-hs.
diabetic skin care q.d. a.m.
diabetic foot care q.d. 9 p.m.

FIGURE 12. Abbreviated care plan for Mrs. Smith.

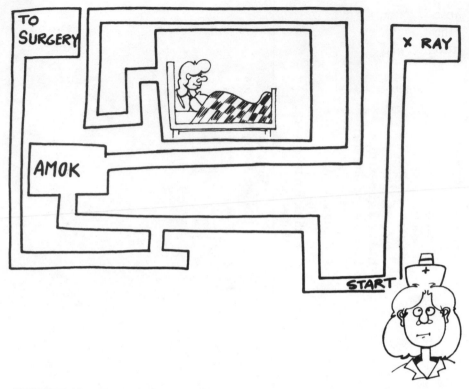

FIGURE 13.   Even the best laid plans sometimes run amok.

GIVING NURSING CARE

At last! The nurse now has a plan which will structure the care which she gives to the patient. She can now proceed to give the nursing care as planned. Even though the nurse has developed a care plan with great effort, occasionally (and in the hospital it seems to be the rule), situations occur which interfere with implementing the plan. The patient may be scheduled for emergency surgery. A patient may be in great pain which alters priorities. Visitors may arrive and the patient is eager to spend time with them. In each case the nurse may be unable to implement the care plan without making some modifications.

CONTINUING DATA COLLECTION

Throughout the process of implementation the nurse continues to collect data. As the patient's condition changes, the data base changes, subsequently requiring revising and updating of the care plan. Data gathered while giving nursing care may also be used as evidence for evaluation of goal achievement, which will be discussed in the next chapter.

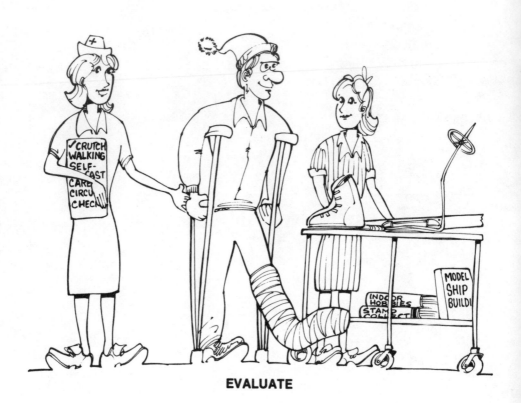

EVALUATE

CHAPTER 4

Evaluation

Evaluation is the last chapter and the final step in the nursing process. There are two parts to evaluation: evaluation of goal achievement and reassessment of the care plan.

$$\text{Evaluation} = \frac{\text{Evaluation of}}{\text{Goal Achievement}} + \frac{\text{Reassessment}}{\text{of Care Plan}}$$

EVALUATION OF GOAL ACHIEVEMENT

The purpose of evaluation is to decide if the goal in the care plan has been achieved. The goal is evaluated at the time or date specified in the goal statement. While giving patient care, the nurse is continuously collecting new data about the patient. Some of this data will be used for evaluation of goal achievement. When evaluating goal achievement, the nurse returns to the goal statement in the care plan. What was the specific patient behavior stated in the goal? Was the patient able to perform the behavior by the time allowed in the goal statement? The answers to these two questions are the basis for an evaluation of goal achievement.

The only thing that is evaluated is the patient's ability to perform the behavior described in the goal statement on the care plan. Nursing actions are not evaluated at this point and should not be part of the evaluation statement. Effectiveness of the nursing actions, orders, and teaching plans will be examined during reassessment of the care plan. The nurse may have given the world's fastest bed bath, but that is not important for evaluating goal achievement. If the goal was to have the patient relax and sleep for several hours, the nurse evaluates the patient's behavior. Did the patient sleep for several hours? The skill with which a nurse performs various procedures is important and will affect goal achievement. However, when writing an evaluative statement, it is the patient's behavior that is assessed. The outcome of nursing care in the form of changed patient behavior is the focus of goal evaluation.

There are two parts to an evaluative statement: a decision on how well the goal was achieved, and the patient data or behavior which support this decision. The nurse has three alternatives when deciding how well a goal was met: (1) goal met, (2) goal partially met, and (3) goal not met.

	Goal Met	
Evaluative Statement =	Goal Partially Met	+ Patient Behavior as Evidence
	Goal Not Met	

If the patient was able to demonstrate the behavior by the specific time or date in the goal statement, the goal was met. If the patient was able to demonstrate the behavior but not as well as the nurse had specified in the goal statement, the goal was partially met. If the patient was unable or unwilling to perform the behavior at all, the goal was not met. For example:

Goal Statement: Patient will walk length of hall and back by 2/7.
Goal Evaluation (done on 2/7 or earlier);
    Goal achieved; patient walked length of hall and back.
    Goal partially achieved; patient walked length of hall but too
        tired to walk back.
    Goal not achieved; patient refused to walk.
    Goal not achieved; patient unable to bear his own weight.
Goal Statement: 2/7 Decubitus ulcer (bedsore) will be healed in 1
    month.
Goal Evaluation (done on 3/7 or earlier):
    Goal met; decubitus ulcer healed.
    Goal partially met; decubitus ulcer still present but is 1/2 the size
        and dry.
    Goal not met; decubitus ulcer broken open and draining.
Goal Statement: After finishing Chapter 4, the student will state

this nursing process book is the most interesting book ever read.
Goal Evaluation (done when the student finishes Chapter 4):
Goal met; student stated this book was the most interesting book
she ever read and asked for an *A* in the course.
Goal partially met; student said this book was about as interest-
ing as any other course books, and asked for a *C* in the course.
Goal not met; student lost book and asked for a class withdrawal
slip.

If the patient problem has been resolved, the nurse indicates on the
care plan that the goal has been achieved. This must be documented according to the institutional requirements but should include the signa-
ture of the nurse completing the evaluation. However, the patient problem identified in the nursing diagnosis may or may not be resolved when
the related goal is achieved. If the problem still exists, even though the
goal was met, the nurse begins reassessment. If the goal is only partially
met or not met, reassessment must always be done.

We shall now return to the patient example, Mrs. Smith, and take a
look at her nursing care plan worksheet with the goal evaluations in-
serted.

NURSING CARE PLAN WORKSHEET   PATIENT: Mrs. Smith

Goals	*Evaluation*
1. Understanding of self-care needs associated with diabetes as evidenced by performing the following before discharge.	
a. Short-term: Planning a 3-day menu for family which meets diabetic diet requirements. Long-term: Prevention of severe hyperglycemia (4 + urine glucose or 2%) after discharge from hospital.	a. Short-term: Goal met 11/13. Dietician reported patient able to plan 3-day menu meeting diabetic diet requirements. Long-term: Goal not evaluated. Referred to public health nurse for follow-up visits.
b. Listing signs and symptoms of hyperglycemia and hypoglycemia.	b. Goal partially met 11/15. Patient lists hypoglycemia signs and symptoms. Confused on hyperglycemia.

NURSING CARE PLAN WORKSHEET(Cont.)

Goals	Evaluation
Explaining actions to take for hyperglycemia and hypoglycemia.	Goal met. Patient stated appropriate actions to deal with hyperglycemia and hypoglycemia 11/12.
c. Correctly performing diabetic urine testing.	c. Goal met. Correctly tested urine q.i.d. × 2 d. 11/13–14.
d. Correctly performing diabetic foot care.	d. Goal met. Performed foot care correctly × 2.
e. Absence of skin infections during hospitalization and after discharge; demonstrating diabetic skin care.	e. Goal partially met. No skin infections occurred during hospitalization. Referred to public health nurse for follow-up visits. Demonstrated appropriate skin care.
f. Demonstrating competence in self-administration of oral hypoglycemic medication.	f. Goal met. Competent self-administration of Diabinase 0.250 gm. q.d. × 3 d. 11/15.
g. Correctly explaining how to cope with short-term illness and manage her diabetes.	g. Goal not met. Patient says she rarely is ill and doesn't feel diabetes will be affected. 11/15.
h. Purchasing medic alert tag.	h. Goal met. Medic alert tag for diabetes purchased through hospital. 11/13.
2. Fear of diabetic complications to be based on verbalization of accurate data regarding progress and complications of adult onset diabetes millitus by 11/10.	2. Goal met. Patient discussed realistic diabetic complications and prevention.
3. Verbalizations of feelings related to diabetes indicating positive self-concept by 11/12.	3. Goal not met. Patient feels anger over diagnosed diabetic condition. Feels if she had controlled her weight better in the past she could have prevented it.

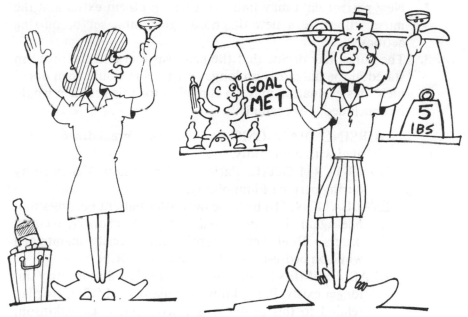

FIGURE 14.   Goal met—congratulations!

REASSESSMENT OF CARE PLAN

REASSESSMENT

The process of changing or eliminating previous nursing diagnoses, goals, and actions based on new patient data.

The process of reassessment follows goal evaluation. Reassessment data may come from various sources. The nurse gathers most of the new data while giving direct patient care. This new data may be used as evidence to evaluate goal achievement and may indicate a need for revision of the existing care plan.

There may be several outcomes when care plans are reassessed.

1.   Priorities may change and problems already identified in the nursing diagnosis may have to be dealt with in a different order.

2. New patient data may indicate a new problem exists and the nurse will write a new diagnosis, goal, and set of nursing actions.
3. The nurse may decide that the goal was met and the problem stated in the diagnosis no longer exists. She would then document this evaluation and the care plan for this problem would be concluded. For example:

> NURSING DIAGNOSIS: Prone to skin breakdown associated with immobility.
>
> LONG-TERM GOAL: Patient will maintain skin integrity during period of immobility.
>
> EVALUATION: (To be done only after patient becomes mobile again, i.e., improved condition, changed medical orders.) Goal met; patient's skin integrity maintained while on bedrest. 11/13. L. Atkinson, R.N.
>
> REASSESSMENT: Problem related to immobility no longer exists. Patient now ambulatory. 11/13: Care plan related to this problem is discontinued. L. Atkinson, R.N.

4. The nurse may decide that the goal was met but the problem still exists. She would then change the goal and/or nursing actions and continue to work with the patient to alleviate or lessen the problem. This is the case when progressive short-term goals are being used to reach a long-term goal. Reassessment involves writing the next progressive goal and the accompanying nursing actions to replace the goal which was just met. Reassessment would end only if the long-term goal was met and totally eliminated the problem identified in the nursing diagnosis.
5. The nurse may decide that the goal was not met or only partially met. There are several reasons why a goal may not have been met and reassessment is necessary to identify and hopefully to correct the unsuccessful plan.
    a. The diagnosis from which the goal was derived may have been inaccurate and require correcting.
    b. The diagnosis may have been accurate, but the goal proved to be unrealistic for the patient's capabilities. The nurse would then revise the goal and actions as necessary.
    c. If both the diagnosis and goal were appropriate, the nursing actions may not have been the best way of reaching the

goal. Reassessment would then involve seeking more effective nursing actions and changing the care plan.

d. The diagnosis, goal, and nursing actions may have been appropriate, but hospital circumstances changed, or the patient's condition changed, or new medical orders were written in conflict with the nursing care plan. All of these
changes would require reassessment of the entire plan to
make it appropriate to the patient's current status.

The Kardex care plan should reflect the updated care plan developed
through the process of evaluation and reassessment. Short-term goals
dealt with during a nurse's 8-hour shift should be evaluated and reassessed. Current progressive short-term goals may be written on the care
plan before a nurse ends her 8-hour shift so the next shift will begin
work with an updated care plan.

Evaluation and reassessment help the nurse develop the skill of
writing realistic and effective care plans for dealing with patient problems. Evaluation of goal achievement gives the nurse the feedback necessary to determine if the care plan was effective in eliminating, lessening, or preventing the patient's problems. When the plan is successful,
the nurse adds to a repertoire of nursing actions and goals which can be
utilized for similar problems in future situations. If the plan fails, the

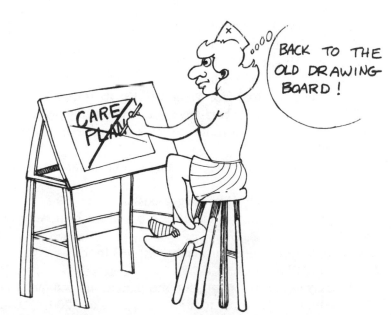

FIGURE 15.   Reassessment may lead to revision of the existing care plan.

nurse can try to assess what went wrong and correct the plan before using a similar approach with another patient.

SOAP charting may be used to document progress toward goal
achievement or to document evaluation and reassessment. Traditional
narrative nurses' notes are another form that this documentation may
take. The SOAPIE(R) charting format might be most appropriately utilized as a summative note on the diagnosed problem and its resolution.
Reassessment (R) of the plan is used in the SOAPIER format to include
documentation of new data, diagnoses, goals, and actions. The next example illustrates possible ways of documenting a plan of care dealing
with a nursing diagnosis of "overweight."

NURSING DIAGNOSIS: Overweight, by approximately 76 lb for
   height.
NURSING GOALS:
   Long-term: Weight of 130 lb by 9/30. (Patient's goal)
   Short-term:
      Weight of 201 lb by 1/14.
      Weight of 199 lb by 1/21.
      Weight of 197 lb by 1/28.
      (2 lb per week average weight loss)
EVALUATION:
   Short-term goal —
      Goal met. Weight of 201 lb 1/14.
      Goal met. Weight of 199 lb 1/21.
      Goal met. Weight of 197 lb 1/28.
      Goal met. Weight of 195 lb 2/4.
   Long-term goal — Goal met. Weight of 128 lb 9/30.
REASSESSMENT: *After short-term goal* – Continue plan. Patient
   is losing weight. Progress to next week's weight goal. Problem of
   "overweight" still exists.
REASSESSMENT: *After long-term goal* – Patient has reached
   end-goal weight.
   Problem of "overweight" no longer exists.
   New diagnosis: Prone to weight gain based on history of over-
   weight.
   New Goal: Maintain current weight within 3 lb for 1 yr.
   New Nursing Plan:
     1. Weekly weigh-in 2× mo, ×6 mo then q. mo ×6 mo.
     2. Gradually add food to diet until intake 1200–1500 cal.
       per d.

3. Encourage *daily* weight monitoring at home with diet adjusted on daily basis to maintain weight.
4. Discuss continuing with exercise program of walking 2 miles q.d.

DOCUMENTATION: Short-term goal. SOAP Format

S . "I'm really feeling good. I've dropped another size. I'm a size 14 this week."

O . Weight 171 lb 4/29. BP 110/70, P 83, R 16.

A . Goal for 4/29 is met. Patient continues to lose weight on 900 cal. reduction diet. Patient is still overweight, approx. 10 lb from desired weight for height.

P . Weight of 169 lb by 5/6 is new goal. Continue reduction diet, exercise program and weekly check-ups.

DOCUMENTATION: Long-term goal SOAPIER Format.

S . "I can't believe I did it. I really feel good. I'm going out shopping for size 10 clothes when I leave here."

O . Weight 128 lb 9/30. BP 112/74, P 82, R 18, Hgb 12.4.

A . Long-term goal met. Patient has attained desired weight. No longer overweight. Problem resolved. 9/30.

P . Discontinue 900 cal. reduction diet. Gradually add foods to 1200–1500 cal. intake.

I . This patient has maintained a 9 mo program of exercise (walking 2 mi per day), 900 cal. reduction diet, and weekly checkups to monitor weight loss and physical health. Hgb monitored q. mo, V.S. q. wk remained normal.

E . Goal met. Patient no longer overweight. Normal weight for height attained. 9/30.

R . Patient may be prone to rapid weight gain with termination of reduction program. Continue to monitor q. 2 wk ×6 mo and then monthly ×6 mo. Encourage exercise and *daily* weight monitoring with diet of 1200–1500 cal. Drop to 900 cal. if 3 lbs or more gained until that weight is lost.

The following is Mrs. Smith's nursing care plan worksheet showing reassessment. Figure 16 shows the abbreviated form of the care plan as it might be written by a staff nurse.

REASSESSMENT

NURSING CARE PLAN WORKSHEET   PATIENT: Mrs. Smith

New Goals	New Actions
1. Describes signs/symptoms of hyperglycemia by 11/30.	1. a. Referred to public health nurse. b. Suggest wallet size card with signs/symptoms of hyper/hypoglycemia.
2. Mrs. Smith will consistently wear medic alert tag.	2. Referred to public health nurse for evaluation (medic alert tag ordered and should be delivered in 2 weeks).
3. Verbalizations indicating resolution of anger and guilt associated with being diagnosed a diabetic by 12/30.	3. a. Referred to public health nurse. b. Encourage communication related to feelings of being dx. a diabetic. c. Share feelings of other people who are newly diagnosed diabetics relating to normal grieving for "lost health."

BIBLIOGRAPHY

Brunner, L. S., and Suddarth, D. S. (1975). *Textbook of Medical-Surgical Nursing*, Third Edition. J. B. Lippincott Co., Inc., Philadelphia.

Campbell, C. (1978). *Nursing Diagnosis and Intervention in Nursing Practice.* John Wiley and Sons, Inc., New York.

Dugas, B. W. (1977). *Introduction to Patient Care*, Third Edition. W. B. Saunders Co., Philadelphia.

Little, D. E., and Carnevali, D. L. (1976). *Nursing Care Planning*, Second Edition. L. B. Lippincott Co., Philadelphia.

Mager, R. F. (1962). *Preparing Instructional Objectives.* Fearon Pub., Inc., Palo Alto, CA.

Managing Diabetics Properly (1977). Intermed Communications Inc., Horshan, PA.

Marriner, A. (1975). *The Nursing Process.* C. V. Mosby Co., St. Louis, MO.

Rehman, J. E. (1976). Writing Patient Care Plans: A Reference Guide For Nurses, Professional Lecture Series, Inc., San Diego, CA.

Wolff, L., Weitzel, W. H., and Fuerst, E. V. (1979). *Fundamentals of Nursing*, Sixth Edition. J. B. Lippincott Co., Inc., Philadelphia.

Yura, H., and Walsh, M. (1978). *The Nursing Process: Assessing Planning, Implementation, Evaluation*, Third Edition. Appleton-Century-Crofts, New York.

ABBREVIATED CARE PLAN

Admitted: 11/6
Discharged: 11/16

PATIENT: Mrs. Smith

Nursing Diagnosis	Goals		Date taught	Planned Action	Evaluation
11/9 Inadeq. info./ diabetes.	Understanding of self-care needs associated c̄ diabetes by discharge. Pt. to demonstrate:			1. Assess knowledge and learning readiness.	
Prone to hyperglycemia related to family and personal eating patterns.	a. Short-term: 3-day menu planning. Long-term: Prevention of 4+/2% urine glucose after discharge.		11/12 *D. Smith R.P.*	2. Teaching plan to incorporate all of specific goals. 3. Dietetic referral 11/10. 4. Provide references on diabetes when she is ready.	a. Short-term: 11/14 Goal met. Planned 3-day menu. Long-term (not eval.) *D. Smith, R.N.* b. 11/16 Goal partially met. Pt. confused about signs of hypoglycemia.
	b. Info of signs/symptoms and remedy for hyper/ hypoglycemia.		11/11 *K. Roy R.N.*	5. Public health referral for follow-up evaluation.	*K. Roy R.N.* c.-e. 11/15 Goals met. Demonstrated: D/U, diabetic foot care and skin care. No skin infec.
Prone to skin infec./diabetes and overweight.	c. Diabetic urine testing. d. Diabetic foot care. e. Diabetic skin care; absence of skin infec.		11/10 *J. June R.N.* 11/11 *K. Roy R.N.* 11/10 *J. June R.N.*		*K. Roy R.N.*

			Nursing orders	Evaluation
Fears possible complications of diabetes.	f. Self-administration of meds.	11/11 *K. Roy, R.N.*	1. Individualized teaching plan.	f. 11/16 Goal met. Administered own meds correctly ×3 d. *K. Roy, R.N.*
	g. Info. for coping c̄ short-term illness.	11/13 *O. Adams, R.N.*	2. Family conference—feelings/concerns.	g. 11/16 Goal not met. Pt. feels goal not applicable. *K. Roy, R.N.*
	h. Purchase of medic alert tag.	11/13 *Adams, R.N.*	3. Offer community support groups.	h. 11/13 Goal met. Purchased medic alert tag. *Adams, R.N.*
Altered body image/diabetes.	Fears of complications based on accurate data by 11/12.		1. Assess reaction to dx.	11/12 Goal met. Pt. discussed realistic complications and prevention. *Adams, R.N.*
	Verbalizations of positive self-image by 11/12.		2. Discuss possible grief response.	11/12 Goal not met. Pt. expressed anger and guilt related to dx. *Adams, R.N.*
			3. Discuss family reactions.	
			4. Realistic limitations—abilities focus.	

Nursing Orders/Tx.	Medications
diabetic urines q.i.d. 6-11-4-hs. diabetic skin care q.d. a.m. diabetic foot care q.d. 9 p.m.	Diabinase 250 mg q.d. 7 a.m.

FIGURE 16. Abbreviated care plan for Mrs. Smith, with evaluations.

Sample Nursing Care Plans

1. **Infant:**   Cleft Lip Repair
2. **Toddler:**   Viral Croup
3. **Preschool:**   Myringotomy Tubes
4. **School Age:**   Seizure
5. **School Age:**   Broken Arm
6. **Adolescent:**   Motorcycle Accident
7. **Early Adult:**   Obstetrics
8. **Middle Adult:** Breast Cancer
9. **Middle Adult:** Heart Attack
10. **Senior Adult:** Cataract Surgery
11. **Senior Adult:** Depression

NURSING CARE PLAN #1

Data Collection	*Data Organization*
	Growth and development

Data Collection

1. 2-wk-old infant girl
2. Admitted for repair of unilateral cleft lip 1/5
3. Surgical repair of cleft done 1/6
4. Infant 10-h. post-op
5. Arm restraints–prevent elbows from bending
6. Infant has taken 1 oz of formula c̄ Asepto syringe and rubber tubing since surgery
7. Patient on I and O recordings
8. No nipple feedings/no pacifier by doctor's order
9. Suture line on lip cleaned with H_2O_2 p.r.n.
10. Antibiotic ointment to suture line following feedings
11. Infant crying frequently
12. Mother in room with baby

Data Organization

Growth and development
1, 12
Maslow
Physical
2–4, 6, 7, 9, 10
Safety/security
5, 8, 11, 12
Love/belonging
12
Self-esteem
Self-actualization

INFANT: CLEFT LIP REPAIR

Nursing Diagnoses

1. Prone to feeding problems related to surgery and unnatural feeding method (data: 2, 3, 6, 8)
2. Prone to trauma to suture line related to frustration of restraints and denial of sucking needs (data: 2, 3, 5, 8, 11)
3. Prone to infection related to surgical lip repair (data: 3, 9, 10)

Goals

1. Oral intake of 18 oz or more per day, during hospitalization.

2. Minimal trauma to suture line as evidenced by little or no crying during next 24 h. 1/5

3. Patient will show no signs of infection of lip during hospital stay.

NURSING CARE PLAN #1 (Cont.)

Planned Actions	*Rationale*
1. a. Hold infant upright for all feedings.	**1. a.** Gravity assists formula into stomach.
b. Feed slowly with Asepto syringe c̄ 1½ ″ rubber catheter extension, 3–4 oz q. 3–4 h.	**b.** Unfamiliar feeding method for infant. Sucking prohibited due to stress it would put on sutures.
c. Frequent bubbling.	**c.** Increased swallowing of air with Asepto.
d. Catheter placed inside of mouth and formula put on top of tongue.	**d.** Prevent attempt at sucking and facilitate swallowing.
e. Hold for 10–15 min following feeding. Encourage parent to hold.	**e.** Safety/security need; calm infant less likely to regurgitate or aspirate feeding.
f. Lay on side following feeding.	**f.** If emesis occurs, side position facilitates drainage.
g. Feed infant on a demand schedule.	**g.** Helps prevent aspiration. Infant crying causes trauma to suture line. Hunger increases ease of feeding.
2. a. Talk with parents about role in holding/touching infant to keep her calm.	**2. a.d.** Crying causes tension on suture line. Facilitate parent/infant bonding.
b. Maintain warmth.	**b.c.d.** Infants' needs for warmth, food, and love are communicated through crying when needs are unmet.
c. Maintain demand feeding pattern.	
d. Pick up infant and cuddle/rock when crying first begins.	
3. a. 3-min handwash before working with baby.	**3. a.** Prevent cross contamination from other patients and staff.
b. Sterile gloves for wound care.	**b.** Prevent microorganism transfer.
c. Clean any drainage from suture line c̄ H₂O₂.	**c.** Crusting and scab formation can cause added scarring.
d. Clean and apply antibiotic ointment to suture line after feeding.	**d.** (Medical order.)
e. Have parents use good handwashing before holding patient.	**e.** Prevent transfer of microorganism by direct contact.

INFANT: CLEFT LIP REPAIR

Evaluation

1. Goal met; intake 18–24 oz/day.
   1/10 *B. Johnson, RN*

2. Goal not met; infant cried for several minutes when blood was drawn by lab. technician.
   1/7 *B. Johnson, RN.*

3. Goal met; no redness, swelling, discharge, or temp. elevation. Infant discharged.
   1/10 *B. Johnson, RN.*

Reassessment

1. None; patient being discharged. Able to take nipple feedings again.

2. Continue goal and actions. New action: Encourage parent to comfort/hold baby following painful procedure.

3. Parents may have questions at home. Provide hosp. phone no. and follow-up clinic appt. slip at discharge.

NURSING CARE PLAN #2

Data Collection

1. David James, age 18 mo.
2. Admitted to intensive care unit with diagnosis of viral croup 2/14
3. Resp. 40/min. with inspiratory stridor
4. T100°℞; P 140
5. Suprasternal retraction on inspiration
6. Nasal flaring present on inspiration
7. Crying when parents not holding or touching him
8. Alert
9. Able to say "Hot" and "Mama"
10. Mother says he understands what is said to him
11. Mother crying on baby's admission
12. IV running at 40 cc/h D$_5$W
13. NPO
14. O$_2$ running at 40%
15. Humidity via croup tent
16. First hospitalization
17. Holds tightly to blanket from home–mother says baby sleeps with it
18. Crying during procedures and examination
19. PCO$_2$ = 48 mm Hg (normal range = 35–45)

Data Organization

Growth and development
1, 9, 10

Maslow
Physical
2–6, 8, 12–15, 19
Safety/security
7, 16–18
Love/belonging
7, 11
Self-esteem
Self-actualization

TODDLER: VIRAL CROUP

Nursing Diagnoses

1. Respiratory distress related to viral croup (data: 2, 3, 5, 6, 19)
2. Fear related to hospitalization (data: 1, 7, 16–18)

Goals

1. Next blood gases in 2 h. will show a decrease in PCO_2 value.
2. Child will not cry during the next 4 h. unless physically hurt.

NURSING CARE PLAN #2 (Cont.)

Planned Actions	*Rationale*
1. **a.** Maintain O_2 at 40%.	1. **a.** Medical order.
b. Check O_2 concentration every ½ h. while in croup tent.	**b.** Keep at ordered concentration.
c. Elevate head of bed 30°–60°.	**c.** Assist respirations–better lung expansion.
d. Encourage parent(s) to sit by bed or get under croup tent to hold/touch baby.	**d.g.h.** Familiar people/things will decrease stress of strange environment. Stress can contribute to respiratory distress.
e. Ensure adequate warmth/do not overheat.	**e.** Cold or heat stress increase metabolic O_2 requirements.
f. Disturb baby as little as possible.	**f.** Respiratory rate increases with excitement and/or fear.
g. Keep blanket within his reach.	
h. Keep parent(s) with baby during procedures.	
2. **a.** Talk to parents about role in calming baby; stay where baby can see them, touch/hold baby inside croup tent, stay with baby during night.	2. **a.b.c.** Familiar people/things will decrease stress of strange environment and provide psychological security.
b. Keep blanket with him at all times.	
c. Have parent(s) assist with procedures.	
d. Explain procedures and equipment to baby in simple terms. Let baby touch equipment before procedure, if possible.	**d.** Minimize fear of unknown.

TODDLER: VIRAL CROUP

Evaluation

1. Goal met; $PCO_2 = 46$ mm Hg. after 2 h.
   2/14 10 p.m. *L. Adams, R.N.*
2. Goal met; baby cried only during venipuncture during last 4 h.
   2/15 12 mn *K Baker. R.N.*

Reassessment

1. Continue goal and nursing actions and reevaluate in 2 more h after next blood gas results.
2. Continue goal and nursing actions and reevaluate in 4 h.
   New Goal: Baby will sleep at least 6 h during the 11 p.m.– 7 a.m. shift.
   Planned Actions: Same as for Goal 2., but add "darken room."

NURSING CARE PLAN #3

Data Collection

1. Matthew Johnson, age 3 yr.
2. Admitted 11/3 for insertion of myringotomy tubes to both ears on 11/4. First hospitalization.
3. Mother states Matthew has had chronic ear infections since infancy.
4. Mother states Matthew has just completed 14 days of Ampicillin therapy.
5. T99 F, P 94, R 28.
6. Weight 34 lb, height 38½ in.
7. Alert, active, playing in playroom.
8. Says he's here to "get my ears fixed so they don't hurt anymore."
9. Mother plans to stay with Matthew overnight.
10. Discharge planned for 11/4 p.m. if uncomplicated post-op progress.
11. No pre-op meds ordered–NPO after 12 mn. 11/4
12. Mother states "I want to go to surgery with him and hold him while they put him under anesthesia."
13. Mother says Matthew still takes an occasional bottle.
14. Brought favorite pillow and stuffed bear to hospital.
15. Mother states she is worried about surgery giving Matthew lots of pain. "I don't know what to do with the tubes in his ears. Can he swim, or take a bath? Will he be able to hear? Does the eardrum grow back or will he always have ear problems?"

Data Organization

Growth and development
  1, 6, 7
Maslow
  Physical
  2–5, 11
  Safety/security
  8–10, 12–14
  Love/belonging
  9, 12, 15
  Self-esteem
  Self-actualization

PRESCHOOL: MYRINGOTOMY TUBES

Nursing Diagnoses	*Goals*
1. Inadequate information related to post-op care of myringotomy tubes (data: 2, 15)	1. Mother will verbalize activity restrictions and care for Matthew before discharge. 11/13
2. Prone to fear related to hospital/surgical experience (data: 1, 2, 15)	2. Matthew will sleep through the night and exhibit little or no crying during hospitalization unless physically hurt.

NURSING CARE PLAN #3 (Cont.)

Planned Actions

1. **a.** Discuss post-op recommendations for Matthew's care with physician.
   b. Assess mother's current understanding of activity restrictions and post-op care.

   c. Talk with parents pre-op regarding son's care at home.
   (1) Swimming restrictions.
   (2) Keeping water out of ears during bathing, hair washing. Special earplugs may be purchased.
   (3) Blowing nose–both nares patent when blowing.
   (4) Child's reactions:
   —groggy post-op;
   —usually no pain at all;
   —little or no discharge;
   —tubes fall out on their own after several months to a year or two. Eardrum seals.
   (5) Care–no special care required
   (6) Notify physician at any sign of ear infection. Foul smelling ear if infected.
   d. Provide written summary of restrictions and care suggestions.
   e. Provide hospital station phone number for questions and follow-up clinic visit.
   f. Review previous evening's teaching on 11/14 after Matthew is stable and prior to discharge.

Rationale

1. **a.** Coordination among health team members.
   b. Beginning teaching at the learner's current level of knowledge aids understanding.

   c. Water will enter inner ear through tubes and cause possible trauma, infection. Increased pressure which occurs when one nare is obstructed when blowing the nose may dislodge tubes. Understanding what will occur may reduce fear and stress of experience for child and family.

   d. Anxiety can interfere with learning. Written material may be resource after disc.
   e. Safety/security need. Emphasis of importance of follow-up clinic visit.
   f. Repetition and clarification of prior teaching improves learning.

PRESCHOOL: MYRINGOTOMY TUBES

Planned Actions	*Rationale*
2. a. Orient Matthew and Mrs. Johnson to the station.	**2. a.** Safety/security needs.
b. Talk with Mrs. Johnson about what she has told Matthew regarding hospitalization and surgery.	**b.c.d.** Safety/security needs. Accurate information will allay unrealistic fears. Familiar surroundings less threatening than unfamiliar surroundings.
c. Explain all procedures and equipment to Matthew and his mother. Terminology/explanation appropriate to 3 yr old. Encourage questions.	
d. Tour of OR, recovery room, and parent's waiting room this p.m.	
e. Notify anesthesiologist of Matthew's admission and mother's desire to hold him during anesthesia induction.	**e.** Meeting Matthew's safety/security needs. Preparation for parent in OR.
f. Discuss sequence of events for tomorrow's surgery with Matthew and Mrs. Johnson this p.m.	**f.** Same as 2.b.
g. Include parents in procedures and care as much as possible.	**g.** Maintaining parenting role for mother. Safety/security and love/belonging needs of child.
h. Provide for physical needs of Mrs. Johnson. Fold out chair next to Matthew's bed for sleep.	**h.** Meeting mother's needs helps her to meet her child's needs.
i. Encourage Mrs. Johnson to follow home bedtime routine.	**i.** Routines very important to pre-school child.
j. Mother and nurse to OR with Matthew in a.m. Take stuffed bear and pillow to recovery room after induction.	**j.** Child and mother's safety/security, love/belonging needs. "Loveys" provide security to pre-school children.

NURSING CARE PLAN #3 (Cont.)

Evaluation   *Reassessment*

1. Goal met. Mrs. Johnson correctly identified restrictions and
   care for Matthew before discharge.
         11/14 *G. Fink, R.N.*
2. Goal met. Matthew fell asleep by
   10 p.m. and slept through the
   night. He remained with his
   mother for anesthesia induction
   and remained calm. Crying
   slightly as he came out of anesthesia. Discharge 5 p.m., 11/14
   to parents. *G. Fink, R.N.*

NURSING CARE PLAN #4

Data Collection

1. 7-yr-old white female admitted to Pediatric Special Care via ER 7:30 a.m. 11/22
2. Diagnosis–grand mal seizures probably related to cerebral palsy.
3. Hx. of mild cerebral palsy. L foot turns in as only sign.
4. Mother states, "She c/o nausea and was breathing funny @ 4 a.m."
5. Child unresponsive to verbal questions, followed by approx. 2 min seizure @ home. Loss of bladder control p̄ seizure.
6. IV phenobarbital and Valium in ER–loading dose.
7. Continuous 7 min seizure in ER–twitching left hand–unresponsive verbally, no loss of bowel/bladder control.
8. Child awake 8 a.m. unable to move left side or respond to painful stimulation left side.
9. Child states, "I'm so sleepy. Where am I? I don't remember an ambulance. Will you stay with me, Mother?"
10. Mother crying and states, "I'm so scared. She's such a bright child. Will she be ok?"
11. IV running to keep open line.
12. Mother states, "This has never happened before . . . I don't know what to do for her . . . should she stay quiet, can she eat?"
13. Mother asks, "Are they going to keep her sedated? Aren't all these drugs bad for her?"
14. Father at home with two siblings–age 9 and 6 yrs.

Data Organization

Growth and development
1, 14
Maslow
Physical
1–8, 11
Safety/security
9, 10, 13
Love/belonging
9, 14
Self-esteem
12
Self-actualization

SCHOOL AGE: SEIZURE

Nursing Diagnoses

1. Prone to injury related to seizures (data: 2, 3, 5, 7, 8)
2. Mother is anxious related to hospitalization and prognosis (data:
   10, 12, 13)

Goals

1. Patient will have no physical injury related to seizures during
   hospitalization.
2. Mother will state accurate de-
   scription of child's condition and
   prognosis by 4 p.m. 11/22

NURSING CARE PLAN #4 (Cont.)

Planned Actions	*Rationale*
1. a. Continuous observation of child.	**1. a.** Physical safety need.
b. Padded side rails up at all times.	**b.c.** Protection should another or repeated seizures occur.
c. Padded tongue blade and airway at bedside.	
d. Vital signs and neuro checks q. 15 min × 8, q. ½ h × 8, q. 1 h × 4.	**d.** Physical safety. Assessment of motor function and verbal responses provides diagnostic data.
e. Orient mother/child.	**e.** Psychological safety. Provide comfortable, secure environment.
2. a. Clarify and repeat info given by physicians to mother.	**2. a.** A person experiencing stress may not accurately comprehend information given.
b. Assess mother's understanding of info.	**b.** Increase data base for further nursing intervention.
c. Correct any misunderstanding and repeat correct info.	**c.** Simple, correct explanations, repeated frequently, are more likely to be understood during stress.
d. Assist mother in explaining info to husband when he arrives.	**d.** Ensure accuracy of info given to father.
e. Explain all procedures done for child.	**e.f.** The frequency of checks and procedures may cause parents unnecessary fear. Understanding procedures may reduce fear.
f. Provide data from vital signs and neurochecks for parents.	
g. Provide and encourage rest opportunities for parents.	**g.** Stress consumes high amounts of physical energy.

SCHOOL AGE: SEIZURE

Evaluation

1. Goal met. No physical injury. No recurrent seizures.

    11/24 ~S. Seiff RN~

2. Goal met. Mother states: "This seizure was related to her CP and we can control it with medication which she may be on for some years."

    11/22 ~S. Seiff RN~

Reassessment

New Data:

1. Transfer to Pediatric Unit. 11/24.

2. Maintenance antiepileptic drug: Phenobarbital 30 mg. q.d. a.m. 40 mg. q.d. h.s.

3. Child states, "I want to go home. There's nothing to do here. Mom, will you stay with me?"

4. Mother states, "How do I take care of her? What if this happens again, or at school? What about sports . . . she's so active."

NURSING CARE PLAN #4 (Cont.)

New Nursing Diagnoses

3. Lack of knowledge related to child's care (new data: 4)

4. Prone to injury if seizures recur p̄ discharge (data: 2, 3, 5, 7, 8)

5. Social isolation related to hospitalization (new data: 3)

New Goals

3. Mother will demonstrate an understanding of child's care related to diagnosis as evidenced by ability to (at time of discharge):
—Correctly administer antiepileptic drug.
—Describe side effects of drug.
—Describe dietary restrictions related to drug.
—Describe home care during seizure, minor illnesses, and use of nonprescription medications.

4. Patient and family will take following safety precautions:
  a. Inform school of diagnosis and emergency actions in event of seizure.
  b. Wear medic alert necklace/bracelet.
  c. Identify activities requiring adult supervision.

5. Patient will play with another child 2 h. by 11/24–4 p.m.

SCHOOL AGE: SEIZURE

New Planned Actions

3. **a.** Assess patient and family understanding of diagnosis.
   b. Clarify and reinforce factual information.

   c. Provide teaching:
   (1) Phenobarbital administration.
   11/24 *JBand, RN.*
   (2) Side effects of Phenobarbital.
   11/24 *JBand, RN.*
   (3) Dietary restrictions.
   11/25 *JBand, RN.*

   (4) Home care. *JBand, RN.*
   11/25

4. **a.** Nurse will offer to assist parents in preparing written summary of condition and safety precautions.
   b. Order selected bands from hospital pharmacy–explain use to child and parents.
   c. Assess child's participation in sports and identify potential dangers which require adult supervision.

New Rationale

3. **a.** Teaching begins at student's level of understanding.
   b. Stress may have interfered with ability to comprehend information.
   c. **(1)** Patient will be discharged on a daily maintenance regimen of phenobarbital.

   (2) Drug may produce rash, learning difficulties, sedation, psychic changes.
   (3) Certain foods alter drug metabolism: ham, bacon, caffeine, chocolate.

   (4) Observe location, duration, progress, tremors, pupils, aura, verbal response, voluntary movement, incontinence. Protect from physical injury by gentle restraint, do not force tongue blade into mouth. Infectious process and some drugs (ASA, cough syrup, nasal sprays) alter phenobarbital levels. Call MD for temp. 100 F or above.

4. **a.** Provide for physical safety need. Written summary ensures accurate, complete referral source.
   b. Patient can begin to wear band as soon as possible.

   c. Swimming, bicycling require adult presence due to high injury potential.

NURSING CARE PLAN #4 (Cont.)

New Planned Actions

5. a. Identify playmate and introduce.
  b. Obtain equipment for shared
  play activity.
  c. Admit roommate as soon as
  possible.

  d. Encourage visit from siblings.

  e. Orient to use of phone.

New Rationale

5. a.b.c. Importance of peer group
in school age child.

  c. Presence of roommate esp. at
  night may help to decrease
  loneliness, fear.
  d. Maintain support system.
  Love and belonging need.
  e. Maintain contact with family
  and friends to decrease social
  isolation.

New Evaluation

3. Goal met. Mother demonstrates
medication administration and
can describe drug side effects, dietary restrictions, and home
care.
   11/25 *J Band, RN.*
4. Goal partially met. Written in-
struction for school provided.
Medic alert tags not yet available—will mail to patient at home
address. Patient and parents
identify activities requiring
supervision. *J Band, RN.*
   11/25 *J Band, RN.*
5. Goal met. Patient played $\bar{c}$ another child and requested move
to be roommates. *J Band, RN.*
   11/24 _____ *J Band, RN.*

NURSING CARE PLAN #5

Data Collection	*Data Organization*

Data Collection

1. 7-yr-old white male.
2. Fractured R arm at elbow after fall from tree.
3. Admitted after closed reduction under general anesthesia at 10 p.m., 4/7.
4. Sibling: sister age 5 yrs at home.
5. Accompanied by both parents.
6. No movement or sensation, thumb and first two fingers, R hand.
7. R arm in traction at right angle.
8. Position: flat on back, small pillow only at head, maintain straight body alignment.
9. Complains of pain in R arm.
10. "Can I go to school tomorrow?"
11. Mother reports child is right-handed.
12. First hospitalization.
13. First separation from family.
14. "I can feed myself with my left hand."

Data Organization

Growth and development
  1, 10
Maslow
  Physical
  2, 3, 6–9, 11
  Safety/security
  5, 11, 12
  Love/belonging
  4, 5, 13
  Self-esteem
  11, 14
  Self-actualization

SCHOOL AGE: BROKEN ARM

Nursing Diagnoses

1. Pain related to fractured R arm (data: 2, 7, 9)

2. Prone to permanent muscle/ nerve damage related to fracture (data: 2, 6, 7)

3. Prone to homesickness related to separation from family (data: 1, 4, 5, 12, 13)

4. Prone to boredom related to confinement of traction (data: 1, 7, 8, 10, 11)

Goals

1. Long-term: Patient will require no pain medication by time of discharge.
   Short-term: Patient will state he feels better ½ h. after administration of pain medication.

2. Long-term: Patient will have full use of R hand within 3 mo. 7/7
   Short-term: Patient will be able to extend, contract, and report sensation in all fingers 4/8.

3. Patient will verbalize feelings related to hospitalization by 4/8.

4. Patient will play with another child 1 h., 3 × per d. 4/8

NURSING CARE PLAN #5 (Cont.)

Planned Actions	*Rationale*
1. a. Assess for pain q. 2 h.–question pt., check vitals and restlessness.	**1. a.** Determine extent of pain by both verbal and nonverbal indicators.
b. Codeine 10 mg IM q. 4 h, p.r.n.	**b.** Potent analgesic.
c. Massage back q. 3 h.	**c.** Backache enhances pain from arm.
d. Smooth and change sheets p.r.n.	**d.** Comfort measure.
2. a. Explain and demonstrate movement check.	**2. a.** Decrease anxiety by understanding what nurse is doing.
b. Assess and record sensation/movement/circulation check of R digits q. 1h × 24 h.	**b.** Increased tissue swelling may decrease circulation resulting in tissue and nerve damage.
c. Request patient specifically to extend fingers.	**c.** Inability to extend fingers is sign of Volkmann's contracture.
d. Notify MD stat. of any reduction in movement or sensation.	**d.** Traction may have to be discontinued if circulation inadequate.
3. a. Ask open-ended questions about separation from family.	**3. a.** Collecting affective data re: potential problem.
b. Follow home bedtime routine.	**b.** Familiar routine enhances security.
c. Explain and encourage unrestricted visiting by family.	**c.d.** Maintaining relationships decreases isolation.
d. Assist in using phone.	
4. a. Introduce patient to roommates.	**4. a.** Assist to initiate relationship.
b. Question re: games he likes to play.	**b.** Assess for interest/skill level.
c. Secure desired games from playroom.	**c.d.** Patient is immobile; play therapeutic for school-age child.
d. Reposition beds and tables to permit play.	
e. Bed curtains open (unless giving care or patient requests closure).	**e.** Decreasing physical isolation results in decreased social isolation.

SCHOOL AGE: BROKEN ARM

Evaluation

1. Goal not met. Patient crying and in pain but says, "No shots."
   4/8 *A Cruz, R.N.*

2. Goal met. Patient able to adduct thumb and two fingers slightly.
   4/8 *A Cruz, R.N.*

3. Goal not met. Patient states to parents: "You can stay or go, but I'm going to sleep!"
   4/8 *A Cruz, R.N.*

4. Goal met. Patient played c̄ roommate for several hours.
   4/8 *A Cruz, R.N.*

Reassessment

1. New Data: Patient refuses injections though in severe pain.
   New Nursing Action: Continue goal. Secure oral pain med order.

2. Continue same goal for next 48 h. 4/10

3. Continue goal. Patient may be homesick later after novelty of hospitalization decreases.

4. New Data: Mother reports patient enjoys reading Super Hero comics.
   New Goal: To provide patient with selected reading materials from portable library c̄ in 24 h. 4/9

NURSING CARE PLAN #6

Data Collection

1. 17-yr-old white male.
2. Driving motorcycle which skidded and overturned. 11/15
3. 15-year-old female passenger.
4. Surgical cleansing under general anesthesia for gravel/sand in facial, arm, leg wounds.
5. Admitted for observation to rule out neurological injury and internal hemorrhage.
6. Scalp lacerations closed; right temporal lobe area of hair shaved and 12 stitches.
7. Parents with son.
8. Parents state, "We never should have given him that cycle."
9. Passenger (female) treated for minor lacerations and released.
10. "I'm not hurt bad. Why do I have to stay here with all of you poking at me?"
11. "Some mess I'm in now; there goes my bike."
12. "What will her parents think? I really wanted them to trust me."
13. "My head! I look awful."
14. Shouts in loud voice, "No, I won't wiggle my toes one more time."
15. Strict bed rest.
16. NPO × 24 h.
17. T 99⁸F, P 92, R 26, BP 110/76.
18. Shouts, "I'm so hungry. Can't you get me some decent food?"
19. Refuses to remain in bed.
20. Up to bathroom: "I can't go in that urinal!"

Data Organization

Growth and development
1

Maslow
Physical
4–6, 14–16
Safety/security
1, 5, 7–11, 19
Love/belonging
3, 7
Self-esteem
3, 5, 8, 10–13, 17–19
Self-actualization

ADOLESCENT: MOTORCYCLE ACCIDENT

Nursing Diagnoses

1. Anger related to hospitalization (data: 10, 14, 15, 18–20)
2. Prone to decreased self-esteem related to accident and hospitalization (data: 2, 5, 11 13)

Goals

1. Patient will verbalize anger and begin to explore reasons 11/16
2. Patient will make two statements of positive self-regard within 48 h. 11/17

NURSING CARE PLAN #6 (Cont.)

Planned Actions	*Rationale*
1. **a.** Approach: nonjudgmental.	1. **a.b.** Encourages verbalization of concerns.
b. Reflect feeling statements to patient, to parents.	
c. Maintain eye contact with patient.	**c.** Shows acceptance and respect.
d. Stay with patient, esp. after verbal outbursts.	**d.** Shows acceptance of anger as legitimate feeling.
e. Acknowledge appropriateness of anger.	**e.** Encourages therapeutic ventilation of feelings.
f. Use open-ended questions to help identify reasons for anger.	**f.** Encourages patient to direct the communication.
g. Explain nec. of procedures.	**g.** Patient more likely to cooperate if understands reason for care.
h. Maximize privacy during care.	**h.** Emphasis on sexual identity during adolescence.
2. **a.** Explain procedures before beginning care.	2. **a.** Knowledge may decrease anxiety.
b. Maximize choices patient can make.	**b.** Adolescent seeks decision making and control of environment.
c. Help patient to maintain grooming and wear own pajamas.	**c.** Adolescent developmental task is self-identity. Body image of increased importance to adolescent.
d. Spend time with patient when no physical care is necessary.	**d.e.** Provide data for positive self-esteem.
e. Verbalize observations of realistic patient strengths.	
f. Provide privacy during phone calls and visiting hours.	**f.** Maintain contact and identity with peer group.

ADOLESCENT: MOTORCYCLE ACCIDENT

Evaluation

1. Goal met. "You're darn right I'm angry. I've really made a mess of a relationship with a person I really care about."

   11/16 *P. Burke, R.N.*

2. Goal not met. Patient beginning to express guilt over pain he had caused his passenger and states, "How can I ever face her again?"

   11/17 *P. Burke, R.N.*

Reassessment

2. Continue goal and actions.

   New action: Assist patient to validate his current perceptions of relationship with his passenger, her parents, and his parents.

NURSING CARE PLAN #7

Data Collection

1. Mrs. Ames, age 26, gravida 1 para 0 (first pregnancy).
2. C-Section delivery 2/4
3. Boy-7 lb 8 oz.
4. 3rd Post-op day
5. Spinal anesthesia for delivery
6. T 98 F, BP 105/70
7. Prenatal BP 100/70–110/80
8. Complaining of "constant, bad headache"
9. Headache worse when patient sits up or stands
10. Headache has been constant since delivery
11. Says she "feels sick to my stomach"
12. Breastfeeding baby.
13. Nipples reddened.
14. Nursing baby 15 min on each breast on demand schedule
15. States, "nipples sore when baby sucks"
16. Breasts enlarged and firm
17. Patient states whole breast is tender.
18. States, "I hope I can be a good mother, but I'm not too sure what to do yet."

Data Organization

Growth and development
1, 3, 18
Maslow
Physical
2, 4–11, 13, 15–17
Safety/security
Love/belonging
3, 12, 14
Self-esteem
18
Self-actualization
18

EARLY ADULT: OBSTETRICS

Nursing Diagnoses	*Goals*
1. Headache related to spinal anesthesia for delivery (data: 2, 4, 5, 8–11)	1. Patient will report that headache is gone within the next 12 hours, while on flat bedrest. 2/7, 9 a.m.
2. Sore nipples related to breast-feeding (data: 12, 13, 15)	2. Patient will report nipple pain is gone during nursing by tomorrow, 2/8, at h.s.
3. Postpartum breast engorgement (data: 12, 16, 17)	3. Breast engorgement resolved by 2/9.

NURSING CARE PLAN #7 (Cont.)

Planned Actions	*Rationale*
1. a. Explain reason for headache.	**1. a.** Knowledge may increase co-operation with bedrest.
b. Encourage bedrest; prone position.	**b.** Reduce pressure of CSF on puncture.
c. Offer pain med p.r.n.	**c.** Chemical reduction of pain.
d. Encourage fluids.	**d.** Adequate hydration.
e. Assist with infant feedings while patient flat in bed.	**e.** Headache and bedrest may make nursing difficult s̄ help.
f. Inform MD.	**f.** Increase MD's data base; new orders?
2. a. Discuss reasons for sore nipples.	**2. a.** Knowing cause helps to understand Tx.
b. Assess for any harmful nipple practices; soap, petroleum products.	**b.d.** To eliminate practices known to damage nipple tissue.
c. Assess for correct breast feeding technique; enc. q. 2–4 h feedings for 10 min per breast.	**c.d.** Incorrect technique can cause nipple damage/pain.
d. Correct any problem in b., c.	
e. Offer pain med p.r.n.	**e.** Chemical reduction of pain.
f. Encourage nipple airing.	**f.** Moistness causes tissue maceration and predisposes to infection.
3. a. Assess for knowledge.	**3. a.b.** Knowing cause helps to understand Tx.
b. Correct or provide information p.r.n.	
c. Encourage feeding every 2-4 h for 10 min per breast.	**c.d.** Promoting breast emptying eliminates cause of engorgement.
d. Encourage night feedings.	
e. Hot packs before every feeding for 10 min.	**e.** Increased circ. decreases tissue edema of breast and reduces engorgement. Improves milk flow.
f. Offer pain med p.r.n.	**f.** Chemical reduction of pain to improve "letdown reflex."

EARLY ADULT: OBSTETRICS

Evaluation	*Reassessment*

Evaluation

1. Goal achieved; patient stated headache gone after pain med while on bedrest and has not recurred for 9 h.

   2/8 *L. atkinson, R.N.*

2. Goal partially met; patient stated nipples still sore during nursing but less than previous day.

   2/8 *L. atkinson, R.N.*

3. Goal met; breasts are soft and patient states tenderness is gone.

   2/9 *L. atkinson, R.N.*

Reassessment

1. New Goal: Patient will report headache has not recurred during remainder of hospitalization.
   New Actions:
   1. Continue bedrest until tomorrow a.m.
   2. If no headache, begin progressive ambulation.
   3. Enc. patient to avoid straining.
   4. Enc. flat position when in bed.

2. Continue goal and actions; evaluate 2/9.

NURSING CARE PLAN #8

Data Collection

1. 35-yr-old white female.
2. Mother of 2½-year-old boy living and well.
3. Admitted 8/27 for biopsy of lump, R breast, upper outer quadrant, which she discovered on self-breast exam.
4. Married 5 yr.
5. Former elementary school teacher.
6. No relatives in this city.
7. Husband is independent businessman "Money isn't a problem."
8. Biopsy positive for cancer, no lymph involvement, confined to tumor in breast.
9. Modified radical mastectomy 8/28
10. Vital signs post-op T 100⁴ F, P 90, R 22, BP 130/76
11. Complaining frequently of pain at incision site
12. Hemovac to incision, patent and draining.
13. Wears glasses–very poor vision.
14. Refuses to look at incision.
15. Asking about clothing–"Nothing will fit me now."
16. "I don't know how Ted is going to be able to look at me."
17. "How can I face my friends."
18. "I might as well throw my tennis racquet away."
19. Crying; talking about friend she had who died of cancer. "I'm afraid they didn't get it all."
20. "I'm afraid my baby won't remember me when I get home. He's so attached to me, I don't know how he'll get along. Nobody cares for him like me."

Data Organization

Growth and development
1, 2, 4, 20

Maslow
Physical
3, 8–13
Safety/security
3, 6, 7, 13, 19
Love/belonging
2, 4, 6, 16, 17, 20
Self-esteem
5, 14–18
Self-actualization

MIDDLE ADULT: BREAST CANCER

Nursing Diagnoses	*Goals*
1. Pain related to surgery (data: 9, 11)	1. Short-term: Patient will state pain has decreased within ½ h. Long-term: Patient will not require pain med at discharge.
2. Prone to permanent muscle weakness in R arm related to surgery (data: 9, 11)	2. Short-term: Patient will brush hair and eat breakfast c̄ R hand by 8/31. Long-term: By discharge, patient will demonstrate four post-mastectomy exercises.
3. Fear related to possible metastasis (data: 8, 9, 19)	3. Patient will give realistic description of her disease and prognosis by time of discharge.
4. Anxiety related to care of son during absence (data: 3, 20)	4. Patient will express confidence that son is being adequately cared for by 4 p.m. 8/29.
5. Prone to depression related to altered body image (data: 9, 14–18)	5. Short-term: Patient will make one positive expression (verbal or non-verbal) of self-worth or ability to do ADL by end of shift. Long-term: By discharge, patient will state three physical activities she plans to resume when condition permits.

NURSING CARE PLAN #8 (Con't)

Planned Actions

1. **a.** Assess pain.

   b. Offer oral or IM pain med.
   c. Offer comfort measures–positioning, massage.
   d. Reassess pain in ½ h. p̄ med.

2. **a.** Explain self-care goal to patient and rationale.

   b. Assess for pain ½ h. ā breakfast and intervene p.r.n.

   c. Position patient comfortably and set up food tray.
   d. Observe patient and assess progress.
   e. Offer hairbrush during a.m. care.
3. **a.** Clarify info given to patient c̄ physician/surgeon.
   b. Assess patient understanding of diagnosis and prognosis.
   c. Correct any misinformation or lack of information patient states.
   d. Use open-ended questions to give opportunity to express fear.

Rationale

1. **a.c.** Anxiety, poor positioning, and poor circulation can contribute to or intensify sensation of pain.

   b. Give patient choices in care to increase sense of control over hospital environment.
   d. Determine effectiveness of analgesics. Most analgesics act within ½ h. of administration.

2. **a.** Patients are more likely to participate in their care when they understand and value the results.

   b. Lower level needs should be met first. Pain interferes with ability and willingness to exercise.

   c.e. Conserve patient's energy for primary task.
   d. Communicates caring and importance of goal. Observation and reinforcement of progress toward goal.
3. **a.** Goal must be congruent with other therapies.
   b. Patient under stress may misinterpret or fail to hear information previously presented.
   c.d. Fear may be unrealistic due to misinformation. Open ended questions encourage patient to verbalize concerns.

MIDDLE ADULT: BREAST CANCER

Planned Actions	*Rationale*
4. a. Talk c̄ patient re: child-care arrangement.	**4. a.** Help to clarify problem for patient and nurse; improved data base.
b. Offer help in telephoning sitter × 3 q.d.	**b.c.** Give patient opportunity to retain mothering role.
c. Help patient write out list of important information for sitter.	
d. Encourage her to talk c̄ husband re: worries.	**d.** Husband can offer support and info regarding progress of son.
5. a. Evaluate a.m. care activities patient able to perform s̄ help.	**5. a.** Success in performing personal care activities will help to meet self-esteem needs.
b. Medicate as nec. prior to activity.	**b.** Lower needs must usually be met before higher level needs.
c. Encourage patient to perform activities appropriate to level of recovery.	**c.d.** Successful experiences encourage patient to attempt more difficult activities.
d. Reflect observations of patient's accomplishments each a.m.	
e. Ask open-ended questions related to effect of surgery on future activities.	**e.** Open-ended questions encourage patient communication. Increased data base.
f. Enc. husband's participation in discussions of feeling, concerns.	**f.** Love and belonging need may be met by husband's participation.

NURSING CARE PLAN #8 (Cont.)

Evaluation

1. Short-term goal met. Patient states, "Much better. Think I'll try walking now." 20 min p̄ med. *S. Lepp, R.N.*
   Long-term goal met. Patient has not requested pain med for past 24 h.
   9/2 *S. Lepp, R.N.*

2. Short-term goal partially met. Patient fed self breakfast but unable to brush hair.
   8/31 *S. Lepp, R.N.*
   Long-term goal met. Patient demonstrated four exercises.
   9/2 *S. Lepp, R.N.*

3. Goal met. Patient verbalized accurate diagnosis and prognosis.
   9/2 *S. Lepp, R.N.*

4. Goal partially met. "I know he's physically ok. but it's not the same as mother being there."
   8/31 *S. Lepp, R.N.*

5. Goal met. "I thought I'd be in bed a week but walking feels good."
   8/31 *S. Lepp, R.N.*
   Goal partially met. "Gardening will be good exercise."
   9/1 *S. Lepp, R.N.*

Reassessment

2. Continue goal and planned actions.

4. New Nursing Diagnosis:
   Loneliness related to separation from child.
   New Goal:
   Brief hospital visit from child.
   9/2
   New Planned Action:
   Suggest brief visit from child. Assist husband in planning visit. Provide for patient rest and comfort prior to visit.

5. Continue goal and planned actions.

NURSING CARE PLAN #9

Data Collection	*Data Organization*
1. 45-yr-old male	*Growth and development*
2. Married, two children (14, 17 yrs).	1, 2
	Maslow
3. Admitted from ER to Intensive Coronary Care Station 7/6.	Physical
4. Diagnosis: probable myocardial infarction (MI).	3, 4, 6–8, 10, 11, 17
5. First hospitalization, no previous heart attack.	Safety/security
	6, 8a., 11, 12, 14, 15, 17a., b.
6. Brother and father c̄ history of MI.	Love/belonging
	2
7. Chest pain began p̄ dinner while watching TV.	Self-esteem
	9, 12, 15, 16, 17a.
8. Admission data:	Self-actualization
	13

1. 45-yr-old male
2. Married, two children (14, 17 yrs).
3. Admitted from ER to Intensive Coronary Care Station 7/6.
4. Diagnosis: probable myocardial infarction (MI).
5. First hospitalization, no previous heart attack.
6. Brother and father c̄ history of MI.
7. Chest pain began p̄ dinner while watching TV.
8. Admission data:
   a. Describes chest pain as "crushing. It felt as if someone put a vise on my chest. It took my breath away. Am I going to die?"
   b. Skin pale, cool, clammy, diaphoretic.
   c. Nauseated "like heart burn."
   d. T 98 F, P 120, R 18, BP 136/80.
   e. Heart sounds clear and regular with occasional premature beat.
   f. Morphine 4 mg IV relieved chest pain in ER.
   g. Elevated cardiac enzymes.
   h. EKG evidences MI.
   i. Monitor shows normal sinus rhythm with occ. premature ventricular contractions.
9. Practicing criminal lawyer, working 50–60 h. per wk.
10. Height 6 ft, weight 220 lb.
11. Normal BP 146/90, pt. states, "My father had high blood pressure too."

MIDDLE ADULT: HEART ATTACK

Data Collection

12. Smokes 1½ pack per day "I've tried to quit but it only makes me nervous."
13. "I've thought about what is really important to me. I'll do whatever I have to."
14. "I have no time to exercise."
15. "I can't live like an invalid. That's no life."
16. "Can you get me a phone. I have to make a few calls that won't wait."
17. MD orders:
    a. Bed rest.
    b. Morphine 1.4 mg IV push as needed to relieve chest pain. Not to exceed 16 mg per h.
    c. Reduce and gradually cease smoking.
    d. Low cholesterol, low sodium, 1,800 calorie weight reduction diet.
18. "What if I have another heart attack? How many of these can a guy take and still make it?"

Data Organization

Nursing Diagnoses

1. Prone to chest pain related to myocardial hypoxia (data: 4, 7, 8)
2. Prone to complications associated c̄ myocardial hypoxia (data: 4, 7, 8)

3. Threatened self-esteem related to MI (data: 1, 2, 4, 6, 15–17)

4. Fear related to MI and possible recurrence (data: 6, 8, 12, 15, 18)

Goals

1. Patient will verbalize no pain during this 8-h. shift. 7/6, 11 p.m.
2. Patient will remain free of complications during hospitalization as evidenced by: stable vital signs, clear heart and lung sounds, normal sinus rhythm.
3. Patient will make two realistic statements regarding ability to safely resume his career. 7/9
4. Patient will identify high-risk factors in current life-style and measures to minimize their effect. 7/11

NURSING CARE PLAN #9 (Con't)

Planned Actions

1. a. Assess patient for pain q. 1 h. using verbal and non-verbal cues.
   b. Explain reasons for pain and continued frequent assessment.

   c. Medicate as required.

2. a. Monitor and report any deviation from baseline data: vital signs, lung/heart sounds, sensorium, cardiac rhythm, urine output, skin temperature, daily weight.
   b. Apply antiembolism stockings.

3. a. Assess patient cognitive/affective level of understanding of MI via reflection and open-ended questions.
   b. Clarify the prognosis and information given by MD.
   c. Discuss concept patient has of self as "invalid."

   d. Reinforce patient's own problem solving skills in dealing with situation.

Rationale

1. a. Pain is indicator of myocardial hypoxia. Pain indicates unmet O_2 need.
   b. Beginning at learner's level of understanding facilitates learning. Understanding rationale enhances patient cooperation in procedures.
   c. (1) Pain increases O_2 demands.
      (2) Determine effect of med.

2. a. Assessment data for indication of physical deterioration.

   b. Aids circulation of venous blood and decreases potential for venostasis.

3. a. Teaching begins at patient's level of understanding.

   b. Patient may have decreased perception under stress.
   c. MI patients can gradually resume work status with varied alterations.
   d. Self-esteem need.

MIDDLE ADULT: HEART ATTACK

Planned Actions

4. a. Approach: nonjudgmental.
   b. Assess patient knowledge of heart disease and contributing factors.
   c. Provide information and clarification.
   d. Using open-ended question, help patient recognize factors in own life.
   e. Using open-ended questions, help patient begin problem solving to reduce risk factors.
   f. Plan family conference when physical status permits to discuss life-style alterations.

Rationale

4. a. Minimize guilt feelings.
   b. Teaching begins at learner's level of understanding.

   c. Improve patient knowledge base for problem solving.
   d.e.f. Participation in developing health care plan enhances cooperation and restores control to individual. Involvement of family will support necessary changes.

Evaluation

1. Goal met. "I haven't had any pain all evening."
   7/6 *M. Knedle, RN*
2. Goal met. Patient remains free of complications during hospitalization.
   7/16 *M. Knedle RN.*
3. Goal met. Patient states, "Maybe I can hire a research assistant to lighten my work." "I'll limit my case load."
   7/9 *M. Knedle RN*
4. Goal partially met. Recognizes: weight factor, high BP, smoking, lack of exercise, overwork, family history. States, "I need to smoke. It helps me think. I can't quit cold turkey." Agrees to weight reduction diet.
   7/11 *M. Knedle, RN.*

Reassessment

1. Continue goal and actions.

4. New Data:
   "I need to smoke. It helps me think. I can't quit cold turkey." New short-term goal: Patient will decrease smoking to one pack/day for 2 wks and consider progressive reduction. 7/25
New Actions:
   1. Check progress q.d.
   2. Reinforce decreased smoking.
   3. Encourage family support.

NURSING CARE PLAN #10

Data Collection

1. 60-yr-old white male.
2. Television repair man.
3. Married 35 yrs; wife visits frequently.
4. First cataract surgery done on L eye 2 yrs ago.
5. Admitted to hospital for cataract surgery on R eye 7/20.
6. 6-h-post-op. 7/21.
7. Says he can see light and dark shapes; cannot see features.
8. Bandage on R eye.
9. "I feel like a baby. I can't do anything for myself!"
10. BP 90/60, P 100, R 20, T 98⁴ F.
11. Admission-BP 130/82, P 88, R 16, T 98⁶ F.
12. Complaining of pain in R eye
13. "I probably won't be able to sleep with this eye hurting like this."
14. Understands medical order to avoid straining, lifting, bending, and lying on R side post-op.
15. "It never hurt like this the first time."
16. MD ordered Demerol 75–100 mg, IM, q. 4 h. held until BP up to 110/70.
17. Took 500 cc fluid orally s̄ problems.
18. Unable to use lens for L eye until 7/22 a.m.

Data Organization

Growth and development
  1–3

Maslow
  Physical
  4–8, 10–12, 15–17
  Safety/security
  5, 7, 13–15, 18
  Love/belonging
  3
  Self-esteem
  2, 5, 7, 9, 18
  Self-actualization

SENIOR ADULT: CATARACT SURGERY

Nursing Diagnoses

1. Lowered blood pressure related to surgery (data: 6, 10, 11, 16)
2. Pain in R eye related to cataract surgery (data: 5, 6, 12, 13, 15, 16)

3. Feelings of helplessness related to loss of vision and activity restrictions (data: 4–7, 14, 18)

Goals

1. Blood pressure will be 110/70 or greater by 8 p.m., 7/21.
2. Patient will state pain in R eye has lessened by h.s., 7/21.

3. Patient will demonstrate use of his bedside control board by 5 p.m. 7/21.

NURSING CARE PLAN #10 (Cont.)

Planned Actions	*Rationale*
1. a. Take and record BP and P q. 1 h. until goal met.	**1. a.** Monitor and document any changes indicating post-op complications.
b. Do not overheat by too many blankets.	**b.** Causes vasodilation and may decrease BP.
c. Apply antiembolism stockings.	**c.** Minimize venous pooling and promote venous return.
d. Encourage fluids.	**d.** Replace lost fluids to increase circ. volume.
e. Encourage bedrest.	**e.** Promote venous return.
f. Notify MD of any decrease in BP.	**f.** Decreased BP may indicate bleeding.
2. a. Assess for factors contributing to pain and eliminate, if possible.	**2. a.** Fear, poor positioning, loneliness can add to perception of pain.
b. Explain reason pain med is being held.	**b.** Assurance that patient's needs are not neglected.
c. Offer minimum dose of pain med p.r.n., when BP above 110/70.	**c.** Physical safety.
d. Offer backrub, radio, and company.	**d.** Distraction/comfort measures may decrease pain sensation and communicate concern.
3. a. Explain goal to patient.	**3. a.** Improves patient motivation if goal valued.
b. Explain control board.	**b.** Cognitive learning.
c. Help patient find and operate controls.	**c.** Practice with feedback necessary with minimal vision.

SENIOR ADULT: CATARACT SURGERY

Evaluation

1. Goal met; BP 110/76 by 8 p.m.
   7/21 *K Adams, RN.*

2. Goal met; pain in R eye reported
   to be greatly reduced after 75 mg
   IM Demerol at 8 p.m.
   7/21 *K Adams, RN.*

3. Goal not met; patient refused to
   try to operate bedside call board.
   States, "I'm too tired to learn
   now."
   7/21 *K Adams, RN.*

Reassessment

1. Maintain goal and actions for
   11–7 shift 7/21. Assess V.S. q.
   2 h.

2. Maintain goal and actions for
   next 24 h.

3. New data: Patient reports he is
   too tired and his eye hurts too
   much to learn how to work control board 5 p.m., 7/21.
   New goal: Patient will demonstrate use of nurse call light before h.s. 7/21.
   New actions:
   1. Pin call light to bed linen
      within patient's reach.
   2. Demonstrate use of light with
      patient's hand.
   3. Have patient repeat #2 unas-
      sisted.

NURSING CARE PLAN #11

Data Collection

1. Fred Morgan, 76-yr-old white male.
2. Retired carpenter.
3. Admitted 2 mo. ago to nursing home; admission voluntary but with encouragement from son; history during past yr of inability to do own ADL.
4. Wife died 1 yr ago, p̄ 45 yrs of marriage to client, states "I can't understand why she had to die, I wish it had been me. It's hard to be the one who's left."
5. One child, a son who is married and has two teenage children at home; son and family live out of state and usually visit client twice a year.
6. Client states about son: "He's busy with his own life. He doesn't have time for me."
7. Oriented to time, person, place.
8. Disheveled appearance: hair uncombed, large stains on sweater, has not shaved for 2 days, sleeps in street clothes unless reminded to remove them.
9. Present wt. 158 lb; admission wt. 169 lb., height 5'11½".
10. States about appetite: "Food just doesn't taste good to me anymore."
11. Complains of early waking, "I used to sleep all night 'till about 6 or 6:30 a.m., lately I wake up at 2 a.m. or 3 a.m. and can't get back to sleep."
12. Except for meals and attending chapel twice weekly, client spends day sitting in his room, looking out the window.

Data Organization

Growth and development
1–5
Physical
3, 8–12, 19–21
Safety/security
3, 7, 17
Love/belonging
4–6
Self-esteem
2, 3, 8, 12–16, 18
Self-actualization

SENIOR ADULT: DEPRESSION

Data Collection

13. When encouraged to attend activities, states: "I'm not interested in anything. I feel so tired; just let me rest."
14. Shows very little facial expression.
15. Client turns head away from nurse each time enters his room.
16. States "I'm no good anymore; what use am I to anyone—I can't do a thing."
17. Denies feeling suicidal, stating: "I'd never do anything like that."
18. Does not initiate conversation; answers questions with brief statements.
19. Complete physical examination by MD 1 yr ago and on admission showed no remarkable physical impairments.
20. T 97.6F, BP 126/80, P 88.
21. Medications: Dalmane (Flurazepam HC1) 15 mg, (O), q h.s., p.r.n., Colace (Dioctyl Na Sufosuccinate), 100 mg, q h.s., p.r.n.
22. States "I miss my house. When you live in a place 30 years, it's hard to move. I had my own fireplace and I was always warm by the fire."

Nursing Diagnosis

1. Anorexia related to feelings of depression (data: 3, 9, 10)

Data Organization

Goals

1. Short-term: Client will gain 1 lb by the end of the week. 1/31
   Long-term: Client's weight will stabilize @ his admission level within 3 mo. 7/1

NURSING CARE PLAN #11 (Cont.)

Nursing Diagnosis

2. Social withdrawal associated with unresolved losses (data: 3, 4, 5, 7, 12–15, 18, 22)

3. Decreased self-esteem related to feelings of worthlessness (data: 2, 3, 6, 8, 16)

4. Prone to suicidal behavior associated with feelings of depression (data: 3–6, 10–18, 22)

Goals

2. Short-term: Client will participate in one new activity by Wednesday, 1/28.
Long-term: Client will initiate contact c̄ another resident @ a time other than meals or planned group activities, within 1 mo. 2/28

3. Short-term: Client will make one positive statement of self-worth within 48 hrs. 1/27

4. Client will deny suicidal plans or ideation throughout stay in nursing home. Evaluate Fridays of each wk.

Planned Actions

1. a. Observe, record, and report I & O.
b. Weigh q a.m.
c. Assess food preferences.

d. Assist client in filling out daily menu.

e. Consult with physician and dietitian regarding between-meal snacks, high calorie and high protein food supplements, possible vitamin supplements.
f. Assist client with hygiene before meals.
g. Encourage client to sit with others in the dining room @ meal times.
2. a. Assess the existence, extent and impact of unresolved losses through use of open-ended and direct questions.

Rationale

1. a.b. Monitor client's progress/evaluate effectiveness of plan.

c. Taking into account client's likes/dislikes may stimulate appetite.
d. Involve client in plan to increase cooperation. Ensure nutritionally balanced meal.
e. Meet nutritional needs of client.

f. Increase psychological and physical readiness to eat.
g. Normal eating situation tends to stimulate appetite.
2. a. Must assess types of unresolved losses and importance to client in order to fully implement plan (Note: elderly frequently have multiple unresolved losses).

SENIOR ADULT: DEPRESSION

Planned Actions

  b. Encourage client to verbalize feelings regarding losses.
  c. Share own observations of client's behavior and seek clarification/confirmation.

  d. Spend 10 min sitting c̄ client b.i.d.; use touch as appropriate; remain c̄ client despite lack of ability to verbalize.
  e. Look over the daily activity calendar c̄ the client and leave a copy in his room; specifically suggest choosing one activity.
  f. Encourage client to sit c̄ others in the dining room @ meal times.
  g. Introduce client to other residents on the unit.

3. a. Assess client's interests through use of open-ended and direct questions.
  b. Encourage patient to verbalize about himself, especially his present feelings.
  c. Continue nursing actions 2.c. and 2.d.
  d. Maximize choices client can make.
  e. Assist c̄ grooming as needed.
  f. Give merited praise and recognition based on specific, accurate observation.

Rationale

  b.c. Increase data base; assist client in developing an awareness of predominant feelings.

  d. Build rapport, develop trust. Convey unconditional acceptance so client is free to express feelings.
  e. Involve client to improve cooperation. Individualize plan to insure its likelihood of success. Decrease isolation.

  f.g. Gradually "repeople" client's life–supply opportunities for development of meaningful interpersonal relationships s̄ overwhelming him. Reinforce sense of belonging.

3. a. Necessary data to guide plan.

  b. Continue assessment. Convey acceptance of client. Increase client awareness of feelings.
  c. Same as 2.c. and 2.d.

  d.e.f. Rebuild self-esteem.

NURSING CARE PLAN #11 (Cont.)

Planned Actions

4. **a.** Be direct in asking client if he is presently suicidal.
   b. Make verbal agreement c̄ client that he will notify nursing staff if feeling out of control or suicidal.
   c. Move client to room closer to nurse's station if feeling suicidal.
   d. Increase frequency of room checks.

   e. Monitor client behavior; observe especially for changes in mood/or levels of energy (be aware of greater risk following these changes).
   f. Alert all staff regarding client's suicidal potential.
   g. Continue nursing action 4. from b.
   h. Permit verbalization of suicidal feelings, do not ignore them or argue c̄ client about them.
   i. Carefully document client behavior and nursing actions.

Rationale

4. **a.** Determine immediate goal for intervention.
   b. Involve client in plan to ensure its success.

   c. Increase nurse's accessibility to client and increase opportunities for observation.
   d. Prevent, interfere with, or interrupt any self-destructive behavior.
   e. Provide data c̄ which to evaluate suicide potential; changes may signal increased suicide risk.

   f. Provide safety and security for client.
   g. Same as 4.b.

   h. Establish trust. Recognize importance of intent.

   i. Ensure consistency of care.

SENIOR ADULT: DEPRESSION

Evaluation

1. Goal not met. Client's weight remained the same.
          1/31 *T. Olson RN*

2. Goal met. Client attended the
   Tuesday evening Bible study
   group, though the group leader
   said client did not contribute to
   the discussion.
          1/28 *T. Olson, RN.*

Reassessment

1. Continue goal and actions;
   change evaluation date for short-
   term goal to 2/7.
   New Data:
       After first refusing to eat
       more than desserts and cof-
       fee, client finished entire meal
       following brief explanation by
       nurse of the importance of a
       balanced diet for good nutri-
       tion.
   New Action:
       1. Reinforce importance of
          balanced diet with brief ex-
          planation.

2. New Data:
   Client states regarding wife's
       death: "You know, I still feel
       kind of stunned . . . it doesn't
       seem real yet . . . I mean, how
       can I face other people with-
       out her?"
   New Nursing Diagnosis:
       Social withdrawal related to
       delayed grief reaction over
       loss of wife.

NURSING CARE PLAN #11 (Cont.)

Evaluation

Reassessment

New Short-term Goal:
   Client will verbalize feelings of
   sorrow caused by the loss of his
   wife within 1 week. 2/7
New Action:
   1. Assist client to review his rela-
      tionship c̄ his wife, including
      shared pleasures and regrets,
      through use of reflection and
      open-ended questions.

3. Goal met. Client states "I used
   to be a pretty good carpenter . . .
   I've always been good @ working with my hands."
         1/27 *T. Olson, R.N.*

3. New Data:
   Client states regarding loss of
      work role: "I still can't get
      used to being so useless . . .
      you know p̄ my wife died I
      sold the house and had to give
      up my workshop and all my
      woodworking tools . . . I used
      to work all day on my proj-
      ects; still would if I had my
      tools."
New Short-term Goal:
   Client will begin woodwork-
   ing project in OT by 2/3.
New Actions:
   1. Consult with occupational
      therapist regarding wood-
      working projects for client.
   2. Discuss working in OT c̄ cli-
      ent and set up a schedule c̄
      him.
   3. Reassess and evaluate client
      self-esteem using direct
      questions.

4. Goal met. Client agreed to seek
   out staff if feeling suicidal or out
   of control, though he continues
   to deny feeling suicidal.
         1/30 *T. Olson. R.N.*

4. Maintain plan.

Index